How To Avoid Rip-Offs At The Dentist

Dr. Carl Kenyon

SOVEREIGN BOOKS *New York*

Published by Sovereign Books
A Simon & Schuster Division of
Gulf & Western Corporation
Simon & Schuster Building
1230 Avenue of the Americas
New York, New York 10020

Designed by Irving Perkins
Art by Dr. Carl Kenyon and
Vantage Art

Manufactured in the United States of America
10   9   8   7   6   5   4   3   2   1

Library of Congress Cataloging in Publication Data

Kenyon, Carl.
    How to avoid rip-offs at the dentist.
    Includes index

    1. Dentistry--Popular works   2. Dentist and patient
    3. Dental care--United States.   I. Title.
RK61.K46   617.6   78-10572
ISBN 0-671-18413-X
ISBN 0-671-18352-4 pbk.

This book is dedicated to the art of dentistry and to all those men and women who have given so much to so many people. Through the tireless efforts of members of the dental profession, millions now enjoy the comforts of natural teeth and the benefits of a healthy mouth.

It is also dedicated to my children, Neil and Elise.

2059115

After you finish reading this book, give it to your dentist.

Contents

Preface

Most dentists practice their profession honestly and well. However, there are those who do not deserve the trust the public places in them. If you are like most people in this country, you have little or no knowledge of the complexities of dentistry. As a concerned professional, I have written this book to acquaint you with the range of services you should expect. I provide guidelines on fair fees to pay for individual services and suggestions on how to avoid unnecessary treatments. In addition, you will find sound, up-to-date information on how to maintain dental hygiene, plus pointers on nutrition to help you maintain good dental health.

If you have insufficient or limited information about the dental profession, you may not recognize a dentist's errors in judgment or be aware of offhand or unprofessional treatment. This book will make you an informed patient-consumer. It will keep you from becoming a victim.

One of your primary concerns is probably fees, which are steadily rising. Present state laws regulating the profession attempt to keep the quality of dentistry at a high level, and for the most part they succeed. However, these laws do not take into account the rapidly growing population in need of dental attention or the growing use of paradental personnel. Dental practice acts in each state should be broadened so that these highly trained people can be permitted to perform auxiliary duties in the office and ultimately foster preventive dentistry; such measures would enable dentists to maintain high standards without raising fees.

In my syndicated column, "The Dental Diary," I have sometimes disagreed with the Dental Society and the organized dental profession. This book is not meant to censure the majority of dentists who serve their patients to the best of their abilities. As a practicing dentist, however, I think it important to educate the public as to what constitutes acceptable dentistry. Any dentist concerned with the well-being of his patients and with better dental practices will be happy to have this book in his reception room.

How to Avoid Rip-Offs at the Dentist

1
Dentistry

The dentist is an unusual professional. He can practice for a lifetime without the dental treatment he offers ever being checked or questioned by anyone. No other professions or businesses have as few checks and balances. The banker has bank examiners who come in unannounced to see how the bank is running its business; the physician is checked by hospital and professional review committees; and the lawyer is in constant contact with his peers in the courtroom.

If the majority of businesses in this country were run as the dental profession has been we would not have the industrial and financial growth we enjoy. Any industry needs competition to make it devise new and better production methods and to make it try to reduce the cost of services.

In American dentistry, the past decade represents the first real period of experimentation in new methods of care delivery for a profession that has changed little over the last five decades. A trend has begun away from solo to group practice, and an increasing recourse to other than the traditional cash-payment method of financing can be noted. The inclusion of dental services in comprehensive health programs is escalating rapidly. The dental profession is also becoming involved in community health planning and in the formation of national health policy.

If dentistry is to meet the growing needs of the American population, the antiquated dental licensure and practice laws in many states must be changed. Paradental personnel must be trained to carry out many of the routine tasks that the dentist is required to perform. Dentists must be relieved from one-on-one treatment of patients, if they are to be expected, as a profession, to treat and educate the majority of the people.

Practice acts and licensure are characteristic of professions and represent the legal basis for their authority. Such legal controls have positive effects in that they assure society that it can expect reasonable protection against harm. However, practice acts and licensure controls also serve to protect the professions themselves by assuring that their occupation is not encroached upon by competitors. Practice acts in particular assure the professions that they can maintain control over their affairs. In this they also represent barriers to change. Some practice acts define the work role of the dentist in a restrictive sense, by limiting the use of dental auxiliaries. Some practice acts have also deterred the development of large dental care delivery systems by limiting the organizational forms they may take.

Dentistry must be freed if it is to grow to meet the public's needs.

THE DENTIST

Some type of dentistry has been practiced as long as man has been on this earth. At first the practice of dentistry involved nothing more than the relief of pain. The next step in the the evolution of dentistry was the replacement of teeth that had been lost. Later dentists began to try to restore teeth in order to prevent and postpone extractions. Today the goals of the profession are to try to maintain natural teeth for the duration of an individual's life and to train individuals of all ages how to properly maintain oral health for life. In addition to the general family dentist, there are now many specialists within the profession.

The Prothodontist

The prothodontist generally has one to two years of special training beyond dental school. His primary responsibility is the replacement of missing teeth, either with a fixed or a removable appliance. The prothodontist not only replaces missing teeth, he also restores them. With patients who have had extensive surgery due to cancer or who have lost areas of the mouth and jaw in accidents he constructs appliances to replace these deficiencies in order to help the patient function as normally as possible.

The Pedodontist

The pedodontist is a dentist whose primary responsibility is to see children, usually from ages three to twelve or until all the adult teeth have erupted into the dental arch. The pedodontist is not only interested in restoring teeth and making the child comfortable, he is also interested in saving the natural teeth. Many pedodontists are trained to perform interceptive orthodontics.

The offices of a pedodontist are usually so designed and maintained that the child is in an atmosphere in which he is much more comfortable than he would be in the office of the nonspecialist. Often, if the parent takes the child to a pedodontist at an early age, he will not develop the fear of dentistry that so many adults experience.

The Oral Pathologist

The oral pathologist is a specialist that most patients never see. There are fewer practitioners in the field of oral pathology than in any other specialty in dentistry; they are usually associated with a large teaching institution, hospital, or medical center. Their primary concern is the study of hard and soft tissues that have been removed from the oral cavity to determine whether they are malignant. The oral pathologist must have two years of extra training after basic dental school, plus he must practice three years under a board qualified pathologist, before he can be qualified to take his own board examinations.

The Endodontist

The endodontist is the dentist who performs root canals. This is the most recent specialty to be recognized by the American Dental Association. Although endodontics, or root canal therapy, has been around for many years, it has only come into its own in the last twenty years. The endodontist has one to two years extra training after dental school. His primary responsibility is to treat the pulp of the teeth in one of several manners so that the teeth can be retained in the dental arch.

The Periodontist

The periodontist deals with the bone, connective tissue, and gum surrounding the teeth. He must have special training, at least two years beyond dental school. Periodontal disease is the most prevalent of all dental diseases. The great majority of adults past thirty years of age have some form of periodontal disease, generally caused by neglect. The periodontist has not only the responsibility of treating all the many ramifications of periodontal disease but also that of training individuals how to care properly for their mouths. Oral-hygiene training is without question the most important aspect of maintaining a healthy mouth and preventing periodontal disease.

The Orthodontist

Most individuals think the orthodontist is a specialist who simply straightens teeth. This is far from the truth; the orthodontist is interested in helping guide proper growth and development of the face and jaws in order to leave the child with a beautiful, healthy smile. Orthodontistry requires two years of training following dental school.

The Oral Surgeon

The oral surgeon deals primarily with the surgical aspects of the oral cavity. There are two types of oral surgeons: (1) exodontists, whose primary concern is the extraction of teeth; (2) oral surgeons who not only remove teeth, but repair fractures, remove tumors, and perform any other surgical procedures involved in the oral cavity and adjacent areas. A board-qualified oral surgeon has from two to four years additional training after dental school and must pass certain examinations to become board-qualified. There are individuals who call themselves surgeons, who are not board-qualified and have no special training. Though many of them are quite proficient, they are not truly oral surgeons.

2

How to Choose
a Dentist

People often choose a dentist by taking the recommendations of friends and neighbors. This is not always the safest method, because people often base their recommendations on the personality of the dentist rather than on the quality of his or her work.

Here are ten questions to ask your friends about their dentist, plus the answers you should receive.

1. Does a filling have to be replaced often?   No

2. Does the dentist ever say you have soft
   teeth?   No

3. Does the dentist or a member of his staff
   instruct you in oral-hygiene training?   Yes

4. Do you have to wait long? Are there
   always many people in the
   reception room?   No

5. Are you always told what the dental
   treatment will cost in advance?   Yes

6. Is the office clean?   Yes

7. Do the dentist and his staff members
   have clean uniforms?   Yes

8. Does the dentist have a posted fee
   schedule?   Yes

9. Does the dentist have a recall system to
   remind you when it is time to come in
   for a checkup?   Yes

10. Does the dentist furnish a leaded shield
    apron for you when he is taking x-rays?   Yes

Ask a specialist, such as an endodontist or a periodontist, to recommend a general dentist. Their specialties in dentistry make them particularly interested in saving teeth and, therefore, prevention oriented. They usually know a general dentist who is like minded.

When you go into the dental office, before you even see the dentist, there will be clues to help you determine whether or not you will receive adequate treatment.

POINTS TO CHECK IN GRADING YOUR DENTIST

- If you have an appointment at a specific time, is the appointment honored? If you wait more than ten to fifteen minutes, you are probably in the office of a dentist who is constantly rushed.

- Is the reception room clean and neat? Are there current magazines and periodicals for you to read? If you find an untidy reception room, crowded with many people who have been waiting for a long period of time, find another dentist.

- Are you asked to fill out a complete dental and medical history? This history is important. The dentist should be informed of any medication you are presently taking or of allergic reactions you might have to any medications or foods, or of any medical condition that might prevent safe dental treatment. If you are not asked for such a history, find another dentist.

- When you are taken into the treatment room, do you find it clean and neat? Are the instruments clean? Is there dust on the light fixtures, furniture, and equipment? Are the personnel (the dental assistant and the dentist himself) clean-cut and are their fingernails and dental smocks clean?

- When the initial examination is made, does the dentist go over your medical and dental history with you?

- Is blood pressure taken? In most instances, the dental patient's blood pressure should be taken by the dentist or one of his assistants, and in many circumstances, the temperature and pulse rate should also be taken.

- Is each tooth examined carefully? Are the gums around each tooth probed with a *periodontal probe?*

- Are the soft tissues—the tongue, the roof of your mouth, and throat—examined? The bite, the way your teeth come together (occlude), and the jaws should be examined. When x-rays are taken, is a leaded apron placed over you to cut down on exposure to radiation?

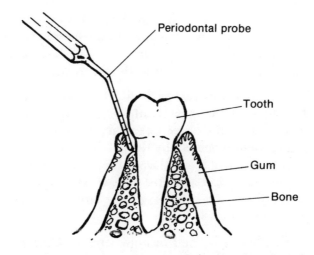

Periodontal probe

Tooth

Gum

Bone

- Are study models made when teeth are missing? This is done by taking an impression of the mouth with impression material from which a stone cast is made.

- If you are an emergency patient, is your urgent complaint attended to first, and are you made comfortable? Are you told by your dentist after he has an opportunity to examine your records and diagnose your x-

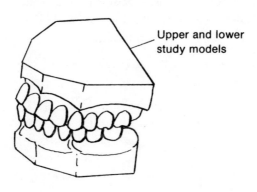

Upper and lower study models

rays that a treatment plan will be presented to you which will explain what is to be done, how long it will take, and exactly what the cost will be? Make sure the dental office will itemize your dental treatment.

• Before a tooth is extracted, is an alternative treatment, such as endodontics (root canal) suggested? Beware of a dentist who is too eager to extract a tooth. (In some instances, dental neglect by the patient or his economic circumstances will mean that extraction is the only possible treatment. Let a dentist extract a tooth only after you completely understand all the circumstances and alternatives.

• Does the dentist himself or one of his staff spend time explaining dental disease prevention techniques, what causes periodontal (gum) disease? Are proper brushing, flossing, and other preventive methods completely demonstrated and explained? If the dentist or one of his office staff spends no time on the subject, find another dentist.

• Does the dentist believe in fluoridation? Does he or his dental hygienist apply fluoride to the teeth?

• Does the dentist or a member of his staff discuss the importance of nutrition to dental health?

3
Fees

A dentist is a businessman as well as a professional. He must be paid for the time he spends in treating a patient or he loses in several ways. He not only loses the cost of the material he has used in treating the patient, and his time, he has also lost because his overhead continues.

With each service in dentistry there should be an equitable fee. It is unlikely that many dental offices' fees will be exactly the same. The fees quoted in this book are a cross section of fees for particular services throughout the country. We have made an effort to demonstrate what is a fair fee for the appropriate service when properly performed.

A dental fee is made up of many factors. For example, if a patient receives a two-surface silver alloy restoration, here is what the patient is paying for: If the dentist is operating on a $30 an hour overhead basis (that is to say it costs him $30 each hour to keep his office doors open, including his utilities, rent, equipment payments, depreciation, insurance, salaries, materials, supplies, and all the things that

13

go to make up overhead), the dentist charges $14 a surface for this two-surface silver alloy restoration, $2 for anesthesia and base. This is $30 and he spends thirty minutes. His fixed overhead of $30 an hour is $15 for thirty minutes. With the remaining $15 he must pay taxes and support his family. If he does this hour by hour each day, he is making approximately $30 an hour for a 240-day year.

All of us know, truthfully, that successful dentists can take in more than $60 an hour ($30 profit). Unfortunately, most people think that all the money the dentist takes in is his to keep. As you can see, this is not true. If one patient defaults, then there is no profit from the other patient for that hour.

INSURANCE

Insurance is becoming an important consideration in dental treatment. Most individuals are now being covered under some type of dental insurance program. However, most of these dental insurance programs pay only for the treatment of the ravages of disease. They pay nothing for and give no consideration at all to what should be a main consideration, and that is *prevention*. All insurance policies should have a provision covering payment for the prevention of dental disease. It is quite foolish and costly for insurance policies to pay only for people who neglect their mouths.

It suggest that any person who has insurance *insist* that there be some payments allowed for prevention. He should be taught how to brush his teeth, use dental floss, use an oral irrigation system, and he should learn the importance of good nutrition. The prevention of dental disease should have a much greater priority than the correction of neglect. Insurance companies would find, I believe, that their cost would be greatly reduced if they would make coverage contingent upon the patient's at least once a year presenting himself to a dentist to have his teeth scaled and cleaned and to be taught the proper methods for taking care of the mouth. If this were included in a policy, I'm quite sure that it would reduce the cost of dental insurance, not only to the patient but to the carrier.

Even with dental insurance, consumers may not be relieved of anxiety about costs. Some dental plans are paying fees based on dentist's charges of several years ago. Other plans claim to pay a fixed percentage of fee schedules, or a fixed percentage of usual and customary fees, or full costs minus a deductible, or 80 percent of full costs minus a deductible, or 80 percent of a schedule that may be only 50 percent of what the dentist charges. And on and on. Premiums increase annually, the employer changes carriers, and new plans with new benefits are introduced.

Moreover, most plans call for prior authorization of treatment plans costing over $100, a device invented by well-intentioned people to prevent overtreatment. The practical result, however, is to put the patient through a series of hoops. He first trots off to the dental office for diagnosis and evaluation. The treatment plan is prepared, and he trots home to await the judgment of some anonymous clerk in his insurance company. After long delays, the dentist is notified that this or that may be done, but this or that may not be done. The dentist, who has had his judgment questioned, proceeds to do what has been authorized. Subsequent treatment requests must be submitted, with time, energy, and money wasted by all parties concerned. If referrals to specialists are required, another pattern of delays and paper shuffling is set in motion.

HOW THE DENTIST AND HIS STAFF TREAT YOU

The dental patient should be treated by the dentist and his staff with courtesy and kindness *always*. Many patients who have used the same dentist for years become close personal friends, but the dentist should treat all patients equally. Fees should be the same for all. The patient's time should not be usurped. If the patient is given an appointment for two o'clock, he should be seen at two o'clock or notified beforehand that he cannot be seen. The patient should always be told exactly what the dentist is going to perform, and educational material such as films, pictures, and slides should be available to inform him. The patient should be aware of the fees involved and exactly what it is going to cost.

No effort should be made to try to sell a patient anything. *The dentist should not be in the business of selling.* The patient does not have the education or the knowledge to understand the different aspects of dentistry, therefore the dentist should not make an attempt to sell a patient something that he does not need.

4
The Dental Examination

THE TEN STEPS IN A GOOD DENTAL
EXAMINATION

1. The oral examination should consist of an examination of all the teeth. Each tooth should be visually observed by the dentist and probed with an instrument called an explorer.

   The portion of the tooth that is visible above the gum line has five sides: the top (occlusal), the outside next to the cheek (buccal), the side next to the tooth in front (mesial), the side of the tooth behind it (distal), and the side next to the tongue (lingual).

2. If a tooth has already received some sort of dental restoration, such as a silver alloy filling, the margins of this filling should be thoroughly examined and check-

17

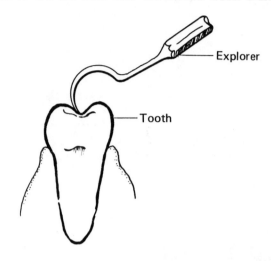

ed to see whether the filling is abnormally worn or in good condition.

3. The number of missing teeth should be noted.

4. The occlusion should be observed, whether it is Class I (normal), Class II (overbite), or Class III (underbite with the lower jaw protruding).

5. The periodontal condition of the teeth should be examined visually with a periodontal probe. Even with the best x-ray examination it is impossible to

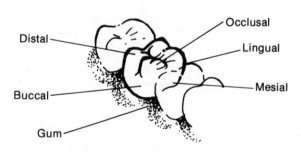

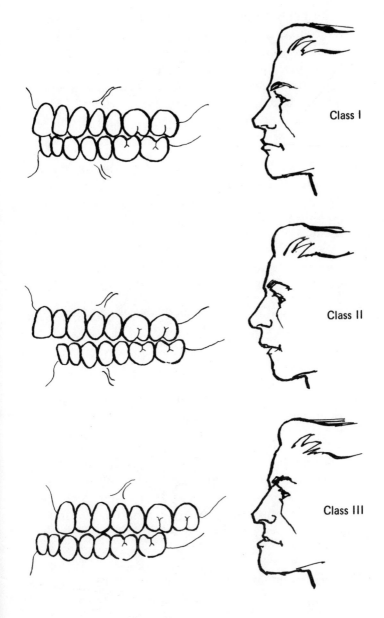

Class I

Class II

Class III

completely determine the condition of the gums and bones that support the teeth. A probe should be used on all sides of the teeth to determine the amount of bone loss and the depth of periodontal pockets, if any, around the teeth. *Periodontal disease is the dental disease most prevalent in adults. A dental examination without the use of a periodontal probe is an incomplete examination.*

6. Conditions of the soft tissue—the cheeks, the area beneath the tongue, each border of the tongue, the throat, the roof of the mouth—should be checked to make sure that no infections, growths, or inflammations are present.

7. The neck and throat should be palpated (felt), to determine if there are any lumps or tender areas.

8. The patient should be checked for bad habits—such as grinding teeth, chewing pencils, and sucking lemons—which can damage otherwise healthy teeth and gums.

9. After the visual examination is completed, a full set of dental x-rays should be taken.

10. The dental examination of many individuals is not complete unless a study model is made from impressions taken of the upper and lower teeth. This is done particularly in those instances in which a number of teeth are missing, or where periodontal conditions exist, or where there is evidence of orthodontic problems.

11. Blood pressure should always be taken.

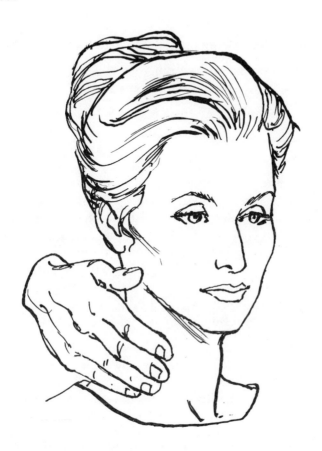

Summary

Be leery of the dentist who simply says, "You have a problem. We'll make you some appointments. Don't worry about it. It will all be taken care of." Unless he is willing to fully explain in a consultation appointment what is going to be done and how much it will cost, find another dentist.

Cost

1. Routine dental examinations range between $5 and $15.

2. Routine dental x-rays range between $10 and $30, depending on the type of x-ray taken.

3. Study models range from $20 to $25.

X-RAYS

X-rays are valuable tools to the dentist and are completely safe when properly used. "Volumes" have been written about dental x-rays and about what dental x-rays will do and will not do. In an up-to-date dental office with modern x-ray equipment, the routine dental x-ray examination is perfectly safe. Most states have laws that require certain amounts of shielding in the x-ray unit, and these x-ray machines must be tested to meet state regulations. There are several things to look for in a dental office:

1. See if the x-ray machine has been tested by the state. If this is the case, there will usually be a certificate displayed by your dentist, much the same as the certificate that is found in elevators to show that the elevator is safe.

2. When dental x-rays are taken by the dentist or the technician, high-speed film should be used. This means the film takes less time for the x-ray machine to expose than ordinary film. Most dentists use high-speed film; ask your dentist if he does. If in doubt, ask to see the box the film comes in.

3. Patients should be draped with a *leaded apron* to protect the body from scatters of radiation. Although most people are exposed to more radiation on a hot,

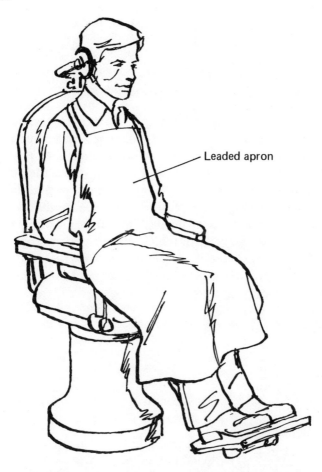

Leaded apron

sunny day than they are when having routine dental x-rays taken, you should still insist on a leaded apron.

Full-mouth x-rays are usually taken every year; cavity-check film and individual films for checking particular areas can and should be taken in the intervals. Many dentists take routine cavity-check films (from two to four

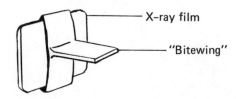

films—called bitewings) every six months, when the patient is in for routine scaling, cleaning, and examination. These x-rays are called bite-wings because they are held in place with a paper tab called a wing, which the patient bites down on. A full-mouth set of x-rays, depending on the dental office, can be from ten to twenty films.

Another type of x-ray used is the Panorex. This involves the use of one large film, which gives a general survey of all the teeth and jaws. Special equipment is required. This x-ray is used by many orthodontists, oral surgeons, and some general practitioners.

Costs

- Single film $1 to $4
- Full-mouth x-rays $10 to $30

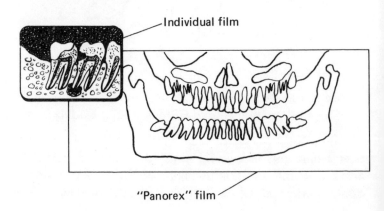

- Cavity-check film $4 to $12
- Panorex $20 to $30
- Cephalometric $20 to $30

THE CONSULTATION (DISCUSSING THE TREATMENT PLAN)

Consultation is an important aspect of dental treatment. A consultation can range from a few minutes with a patient in the ordinary dental treatment room to a meeting in the dentist's office. At this time the dentist and the patient should review the treatment plan. The patient should have the opportunity to ask questions about the recommended treatment. Three major questions should be asked—questions that the dentist should be most readily prepared to answer.

1. What does he plan for the treatment?
   Answer: The treatment plan should be broken down so that the teeth can be discussed individually and in logical sequence. Everything should be explained in such a way that the patient can understand what is going to take place in his mouth.

2. How long is the treatment going to take?
   Answer: When an accurate and concise treatment plan has been prepared, the dentist should be able to tell the patient, within reason, how long each visit will be and how much time between treatment appointments will be required for laboratory work.

3. How much is this going to cost?
   Answer: Exact fixed fees, not approximations, should be determined in advance. These fees should be item-

ized so that the patient knows exactly what he is paying for.

All possible contingencies should be discussed by the dentist. For example, often a badly decayed tooth, after it has been properly prepared and restored, will still require endodontics either following the initial treatment or sometime in the future. The patient should be made aware of this.

Many dentists prepare two treatment plans since dental needs and financial resources can vary from patient to patient. Both treatment plans are presented so that the patient can be the one who makes the decision as to what kind of treatment he desires. For example, a few missing teeth can be replaced in most cases with either a fixed bridge or a removable partial denture. The fixed bridge, simply by the nature of the mechanics and time involved, along with the laboratory expense, costs a great deal more; however, it does have an advantage of being fixed in place. Many individuals can't afford a fixed bridge so they have to take the usually less expensive alternative treatment plan of removable partial dentures.

There should be complete understanding between the dentist and the patient before any treatment is initiated. Within reason, the patient should know exactly what is going to be done in his particular case, how long it will take, what the alternatives are, and what the possibilities are of further treatment in the future.

The importance of routine oral hygiene at home must be stressed; if all the aspects of dental treatment are fully discussed before the start of treatment, most of the problems that occur between dentists and patients can be avoided.

This should not be a time when the dentist makes an

effort to *sell*. His responsibility is to inform, to recommend
to the patient what is best for his particular problem.

Cost

If a dentist takes fifteen to thirty minutes or an hour of
his time to discuss your problems with you, you are
expected to pay for it. The cost of consultation appointments can range from $10 to $30.

THE TREATMENT PLAN

The dentist should give you a copy of the treatment
plan at the start of treatment so that you can review, and
discuss objectively all aspects of the plan and the arrangements with members of your family if necessary. The
terminology used in the plan should be easily understand-
able. If need be, you can consult another dentist. An ethi-
cal, honest dentist is never afraid to have his x-rays,
treatment plan, or patient record sent to another dentist.
Of course, all dentists want to keep *almost* every patient in
their office, but even the best dentist cannot please everybody. In addition to the copy of the treatment plan
made for you, a copy should be kept in your record folder.

Diagnostic skills are required to prepare a treatment
plan, and their acquisition is without question one of the
most important aspects of a dentist's training. If a dentist
doesn't take the time to make as thorough a diagnosis as
possible, then it is impossible for him to construct a treatment program suited to the individual patient. This plan
should be as useful to the dentist as it is to you. Accurately
and conscientiously prepared, it is a blueprint from which
the dentist can carry out his treatment.

Your initial visit to the dentist (other than one caused by

an emergency) should have consisted of the taking a dental and medical history, an adequate oral examination including a periodontal probe, the taking of x-rays, and possibly the casting of study models. From these diagnostic aids, and using his training and experience, the dentist will have determined the treatment plan.

A treatment plan can be a printed form or it can be typed individually for the patient, but it should be in writing. When a thorough, well-prepared treatment plan has been made in advance by your dentist, it not only informs you of what you can expect, but demonstrates that you are in a well-organized office, and that the dentist has a definite plan of how to take care of your dentistry.

One of the things that often reveals a poorly organized dental office and indicates poor dentistry is a dentist who holds the x-rays up to the light and prepares the treatment plan while you are sitting in the dental chair. If the treatment plan is not prepared before you come to the dental office or if it is not in writing (if the dentist simply tells you verbally that it will cost x number of dollars to "fix" your teeth), then make the dentist explain exactly what is going to be done. If you still have confidence in this dentist, make him write down in advance exactly what will be performed. If your dentist will not outline a treatment plan for you in advance, find another dentist.

The dentist who does not use a treatment plan will many times ask, "Well, what are we going to do to you today?" because he has really forgotten what he told you the last time and he is expecting you to remember. A dentist who has a treatment plan knows what is going to be done when he starts the treatment, and as each portion is carried out, it is checked off. This is the organized way to carry out accurate treatment.

FINANCIAL ARRANGEMENTS

You should come to a thorough understanding of the financial arrangements with your dentist. This should be in writing and should be agreed upon before treatment is ever started. Be prepared to pay for your dentistry. This is one of the most difficult aspects of dental care to discuss, because many dentists throughout the world have different policies concerning finance arrangements. Remember, however: *Your dentist is not a banker.* A dentist is a professional, but he is not in the business of lending money. A dentist should not be expected to extend credit for more than thirty days, and then only on a limited basis. If you need to spread your dental payments over a longer period of time, you should arrange it in advance, at a lending institution, such as a bank, credit union and/or savings and loan institution. You can also take advantage of the many financing plans available. Credit cards, including Master Charge and Visa, are accepted in most dental offices. Financing is the business of the banks and credit card companies. It is the dentist's business to take care of your dental needs.

There are various insurance plans available today, with more coming on the scene, that will take care of dental needs. All of these plans are different. Insurance contracts are contracts between the patient and the insurance company. The dentist is a third party. Many patients are under the impression that if they have a dental insurance plan, whatever the dentist charges will be paid by the insurance company. This is far from true.

Unless the dental problem is due to an accident, most plans pay only a portion of the dental fee. If you have an insurance plan, discuss it with your dentist, or with the dentist's secretary or dental business manager prior to your treatment. If you have an insurance plan that requires approval by your insurance company (called a predetermination of benefits), as many do, the dental office can usually determine approximately what you can expect from your dental insurance. The remainder will have to be paid by you. Many insurance companies take months to pay. The dentist should not be asked to carry this burden. If he is willing to wait until the insurance company pays, you will be asked to assign the insurance claim to the dentist and be expected to pay interest, as you would for any other form of credit. Because of the hundreds of different insurance company claim forms, the amount of time it takes to fill out these claims, and the expense to the dentist, many offices will charge for this service. This charge is perfectly justifiable and should be $3 to $5.

Summary

If you go to a dentist and he puts you in a chair and says, "Open," and goes to work without informing you what he is doing, tell him that you would like an opportunity to find out exactly what he plans to do, exactly how long it will take, how many appointments will be necessary, and above all, how much it will cost. If he refuses to do this, or passes over it lightly, or cannot explain exactly what he is going to do and is hedging about the cost, find another dentist.

The dentist's regular and customary fees should be available in writing for the patient to review. Have the dentist explain the work to you, regardless of the amount of dental treatment involved, whether it is one "filling" or a full mouth rehabilitation. He should explain and be willing to put the information in writing. The dentist should have available for you, your x-rays, models of your mouth, drawings, and diagrams so that you can understand exactly what is going to take place.

You should be concerned about what the dentist charges, that it is a fair fee, but you should be more concerned that the fee he is charging is justified by the service to be rendered.

5
The
Dental Hygienist

In Connecticut, in 1907, the laws were changed so that a specially trained person could examine and clean the teeth. This was the recognition of the professional position we now call the dental hygienist. The dental profession was at first slow to recognize the need for hygienists, but today they have become an integral part of the dental office and the profession in all fifty states. Licensing is now required for this most valuable and needed professional auxiliary.

When we speak of dental hygienists we think of women, but more and more today, male dental hygienists are practicing in the United States and throughout the rest of the world. To qualify for a license the dental hygienist must have least two years of college plus training in a two-year program in dental hygiene. The hygienist works under the supervision of a dentist, who is responsible for the services performed.

The hygienist's concern is the prevention of oral disease. He or she assists the dentist in a program of preventive dental care that consists of the following:

1. Oral prophylaxis (scaling and cleaning)

2. Topical fluoride treatments

3. Taking x-rays

4. Discussing health with patients

5. Teaching hygiene and diet control to the patient

The whole field of dentistry today is placing special emphasis on preventive methods, and dental hygiene has become a challenging profession. Through the years, as the science of dentistry continues to develop, the responsibilities of the dental hygienist will expand.

It is not possible to increase the number of dental school graduates enough to keep pace with the rapid increase in the national population and maintain the present high standards of dental education. For this reason, the dental hygienist is an important part of the dental health team. The hygienists with their expanded duties can relieve the dentist in order that he may be of greater service to the patients he sees and may have the opportunity to see more patients in the dental office.

The dental hygienist may have many responsibilities on which the efficiency of a well-organized dental office will depend. The dental office that has a dental hygienist who is conscientious in performing the prophylaxis and in providing the education programs on oral hygiene usually is one that is thorough in its approach to dental care. It cannot be said that all dental offices that have dental hygienists are infallible in their diagnosis and treatment, but for the most part these are the offices that are most likely to give the best dental care.

RECALL SYSTEM

The recall system is handled differently in many dental offices. Some give the patient an appointment three to six months in advance, some send the patients a card, or make a telephone call to the patient. In most offices that have a dental hygienist, the hygienist is responsible for the recall system.

With an adequate recall system the patient is encouraged periodically to have his teeth scaled and cleaned, x-rays taken, and examinations made of all hard and soft tissues in the mouth. Reviewing the patient's oral-hygiene techniques is an important aspect of overall dental care. A dental office that has a good recall system and is meticulous in its work is usually one interested in the patient's dental health care and in saving teeth.

There are several things that should be observed in a routine recall system.

1. Be skeptical of the type of system in which the recall examination takes only about fifteen minutes, no emphasis is placed on how the patient is taking care of his mouth (flossing, brushing, etc.), and the patient is not asked to chew a disclosing tablet to discover how he is brushing his teeth.

2. If you never see the dentist, but simply see the hygienist time after time, this is another indication that the recall system is just a way to get patient flow into the office and increase income.

It takes at least thirty to forty minutes for most hygienists to adequately scale and clean the teeth, to check the patient's oral-hygiene techniques, and to discuss any particular problems that the patient may be having. It is advisable, at the end of the recall, for the patient's mouth to be checked by the dentist. At this time the dentist and hygienist can discuss any weakness found in the patient's daily oral-hygiene techniques. It is not just the recall system that is important, but how the recall system is maintained, and what services are performed once you arrive in the dental office.

2059115

HOW HYGIENISTS ARE PAID

Many hygienists are paid a percentage of the fees that are charged the patients. The more patients they see, the more money they make. A good question to ask your hygienist is how many patients he or she sees a day. If the answer is more than eight to ten patients a day, it is impossible for the hygienist to be doing an adequate job. If your dental hygienist does not do the following, then I would say you need to have a discussion with your dentist, or change dental offices:

1. Spend time on oral-hygiene training

2. Check to see how you are brushing and taking care of your teeth

3. Ask you about your nutritional program

4. Use a periodontal probe around your teeth to see the condition of your gums

Cost

The usual fee for the dental hygienist to perform the services discussed above should be between $10 and $20, not including x-rays.

6
Oral-Hygiene Training

Oral-hygiene training in the dental office is an important aspect of dentistry. Carried out by only a small minority of the profession for many years, it has received more emphasis in the past decade than ever before. In a dental office offering a dental disease prevention program, a patient will be taught what causes tooth decay and periodontal disease and how to use biological stains (disclosing tablets) on the teeth to see where bacteria are accumulating on the patient's teeth. He can see for himself where the plaque is located and what should be removed. Until individuals develop good oral-hygiene programs, they should use these tablets daily.

Some dentists do not use disclosing tablets; instead, they feel that if any blood is seen during brushing or flossing, this means that the patient is not doing an adequate job and must improve his techniques. If blood is apparent, there may be a periodontal problem involved which should receive immediate attention by the dentist. On the other hand, just because your gums don't bleed, don't be misled into believing that you cannot have periodontal disease. You can have a chronic periodontal disease and your gums will not bleed.

Patients should be informed as to the type of toothbrush to use (one with rounded, soft bristles), the best type of toothpaste (abrasive or nonabrasive), the use of toothpicks, the use of oral lavage equipment such as a water pick, and the types of dental flosses that should be used. Proper techniques should be shown to the patient, and the patient should be tested periodically. It should be emphasized again and again to the patient exactly how to take care of his teeth.

Every dental office should provide instruction to train patients to care properly for their mouths. Most dentists today still do not provide this type of service for the patient. A survey was performed among fifteen hundred

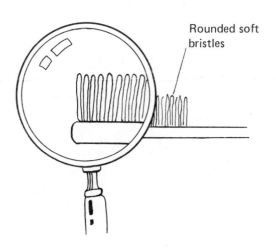

Rounded soft bristles

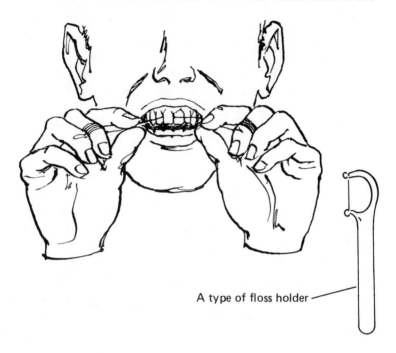

A type of floss holder

general dentists and it was found that 84 percent of them did not offer their patients a systematic instruction program in plaque control or oral-hygiene training. Only 8 percent of those surveyed had such a program in their office.

One of the most disheartening problems that dentists face is that even though many of them have been offering a systematic program good oral-hygiene training for years, they find that most patients are interested when they first tell them about plaque control but, in fact, only 10 percent to 20 percent change their oral-hygiene habits, and 80 percent of these people in a short time go back to the same old method of cleaning their teeth.

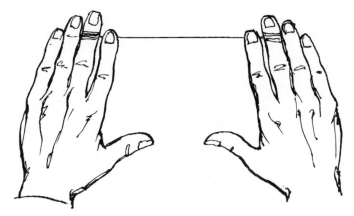

The proper ways to hold floss

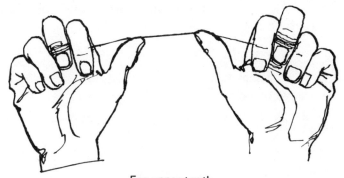

For upper tooth

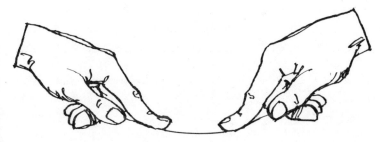

For lower tooth

Most important area to brush

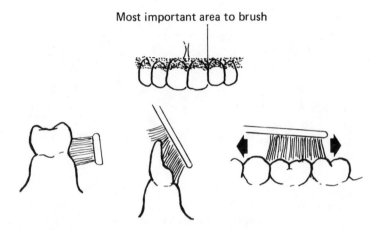

Remember, a good oral-hygiene program should show you the following:

1. How to select the proper type of toothbrush

2. How to select the best type of toothpaste, whether abrasive or nonabrasive

3. How to use toothpicks properly; how to floss properly

4. How to use water lavage equipment (water pick)

5. How to brush and when to brush

6. How to use disclosing tablets or stains that help you see if you are brushing and flossing properly

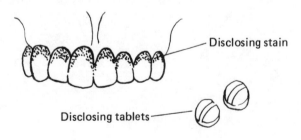

7
Nutrition

Nutrition is an important aspect in total dental health care. The dentist should make you aware of the need for good nutrition, and any extensive dental treatment that does not include at least an outline of good nutrition is not good dental care.

Nutrition that is good for dental health is no different from that necessary for general good health. Recognizing that nutrition is an important aspect of adequate dental care, the dental profession today has placed a great deal of importance on nutrition as part of a complete prevention program. Many dental offices are now counseling their patients on diet and asking the patient to monitor his eating habits by keeping a food diary. While doing this, a person can see how much sugar he is consuming, how often, and in what form. He can then take steps to improve his dental health by changing his eating habits.

Bacteria prefer foods that are high in unstable refined carbohydrates. Since these foods start the production of

41

acid in the plaque, we will call them starter foods. Some samples of starter foods are:

1. Cereals, breads, cakes, pies, cookies, and other pastries

2. Sweetened soft drinks, colas, chocolate milk, and coffee or tea with sugar

3. Jams, jellies, sugars, gums, candies, breath mints, cough drops, and sugar gums

Sugar by itself is not the cause of dental problems, but gum disease and tooth decay are related to dental plaque, a slick colorless film of harmful oral bacteria that constantly forms on the teeth. The combination of the sugar and certain bacteria in the plaque work together to develop acids, which in turn attack the tooth enamel, eventually leading to decay. Natural carbohydrates (fruits, vegetables) are not nearly as damaging as refined carbohydrates.

Natural carbohydrates—for example, apples or oranges —are a sugar that comes in the form of fructose. In order for the body to assimilate fructose, it must be broken down by metabolic action and eventually changed to glucose, which can be absorbed by the cell. The single-cell bacteria that are common in the mouth also assimilate this fructose and break it down to make it glucose. White sugar is in the form of glucose already and the moment that it is taken into the mouth the bacteria assimilate it almost instantly, converting it into harmful acids.

During the period of time when acid is present, some of the tooth surface is dissolved. Once acid has been produced in the plaque, it may be as long as an hour before it is diluted and neutralized by the saliva, even though the food may have been present for only a few moments. A hole can form in the tooth after many acid attacks. When regular meals are eaten, the amount of time that the teeth are exposed to the acid attack can be seen to last for approximately an hour after breakfast, lunch, and dinner. However, let's look at what happens when starter foods are added as between-meal snacks. If you eat breakfast, midmorning snacks, lunch, afternoon snacks, dinner, and bedtime snacks, your teeth are exposed to almost continuous attack from these starter foods. The amount of tooth decay is directly related to the amount of time the tooth is exposed to the acid produced by the bacteria. Repeated exposure to acid will cause cavities to form in your teeth.

Gum disease is also initiated when irritants are formed by the bacteria in the plaque. This process, if unchecked, leads to bleeding gums, loosened teeth, and eventual loss of teeth.

There are many enjoyable snacks that can be substituted for starter foods. Popcorn is an especially good snack food. Other examples are cottage cheese, cheese products, fresh fruits, unsweetened fruit juices, deviled eggs or hard-boiled eggs, luncheon meats or leftover meats, peanuts, carrots, celery sticks, and other nuts and their derivatives. If you chew gum it should be sugarless gum. It is not necessary to completely deprive yourself of all carbohydrates; the most important carbohydrates are unrefined ones, such as fruits and vegetables. The prevention of tooth decay and periodontal disease is an important health concern and it should bear a direct relation to how often you eat starter foods. Any foods that remain in the mouth for long periods of time are more harmful than the ones swallowed immediately. For example, breath mints are probably the most destructive food you can place in your mouth.

One of the natural defenses against acid attack during the day is your saliva, which helps neutralize some of the acid produced by the bacteria. At night, when you are sleeping, you do not have as much saliva as during the day. Consequently, it is most important to have as clean a mouth as possible upon retiring.

Your dentist or dental hygienist will tell you which foods bacteria use to produce harmful acids. They may also recommend the use of fluoride toothpaste. But, remember, it is most important to clean your teeth by brushing and flossing thoroughly each day, for a clean tooth will not decay or have periodontal disease. If your dentist does not (1) discuss the particular nutritional needs for your age group, (2) discuss what you eat, or (3) discuss how you take care of your mouth, then I recommend that you find another dentist.

Six steps that you should understand when selecting food for good dental health:

1. Check the labels of all products to see if sugar has been added. A close look will often reveal hidden sugar in items previously thought to be sugarless (when checking labels remember that sugar may also be listed as corn syrup, sucrose, or dextrose).

2. Stay away from items, such as glazed doughnuts, that are heavily laden in refined sugars. Serve your children a good nutritious breakfast (stay away from the convenience foods, which you will find are usually saturated with sugars).

3. Chewing gum and soft drinks are not necessities of life, but if you must buy them, choose the sugarless gums and diet soft drinks.

4. When preparing snacks for your children, use raw vegetables such as carrots, celery, radishes, tomatoes, cabbage, lettuce, cucumbers, and fresh fruits. Nutri-

tionally, these are much better for you and would certainly be better for your dental health.

5. At a birthday party for children, substitute fresh fruit, or ice cream made with sugar substitutes, for the conventional decorated birthday cake. Also substitute fruit juices, tomato juices, and sugarless soft drinks.

6. Avoid cereals with candy or sugar coatings; when serving cereals to children, use the natural cereals that have no added sugar.

The goal of good nutrition is to provide daily an adequate and well-balanced supply of all nutrients. Fulfillment of the goal requires not only the availability of appropriate, high-quality food but, in addition, the food should be prepared adequately to preserve nutritional values and should be served in a palatable and aesthetic fashion. Proper nutrition is important throughout life. An example of how important proper nutrition is to dentistry is that of the mother's diet during pregnancy. If the mother's diet is deficient in calcium, phosphorous, or vitamin D during pregnancy, this can have an effect on the development of the teeth of the embryo. If these same deficiences (calcium, phosphorous, and vitamin D) are lacking in the diet of a young child, the damage cannot be erased by later addition of these foods to the diet. Chemical composition and the histological integrity of the teeth reflect the nutritional circumstances during mineralization and serve as an adequate picture of the kind of nutritional deficiencies that have occured in the child's life.

Our individual cells are incredible, complex engines, and they are capable of liberating stored chemical energy to do work within the body or surrounding environment. The kind of work varies from one cell to another and covers a multitude of energy transformations. This energy comes from the nutrients that we take into our body; the most effective nutrients can produce the best sources of energy. Whether the energy is expended in movement or exercise, or in energy required for the maturation of cells, what we eat is important. Whereas, the gasoline engine requires gas and oxygen as its sole combustible nutrient, cells not only need fuel as their energy source and oxygen for oxidation, but they also demand a variety of other chemicals to liberate energy and to provide building blocks for body tissue. In addition to needing oxygen as an energy source, cells require:

1. Water

2. One or more polyunsaturated fatty acids

3. At least twenty amino acids

4. Thirteen vitamins

5. Thirteen minerals

Just as a motor stops when all the gasoline has been burned, so do the cells die when the supply of any of these nutrients has been exhausted. The stoppage of one or more of the cellular activities might not be as conspicuous or dramatic as that which would occur in a gasoline engine, but, nonetheless, the end would eventually be the same. Cells faced with metabolic disorder or poor absorption of nutrients behave similarly to a gasoline engine with a dirty carburetor, improper fuel-oxygen mixture, or poor timing. In other words, if you ingest an improper diet, even though you may have a feeling of fullness and satisfaction from eating, the foods that you have eaten may be of no value to the cellular metabolism of your body.

A general guide for good eating habits should stress:

1. Three or more glasses of milk daily for children, smaller glasses for children under nine; four or more glasses of milk for teenagers; and one glass for adults (for adults it should be the nonfat variety). Cheese, ice cream, and other milk products can supply part of the daily milk requirements.

2. Two or more servings of meat daily. Fish, poultry, eggs, cheese, dried beans, peas, or nuts are alternatives. (It is advisable for adults to eat less beef and more fish and poultry.)

3. Fruits and vegetables, four or more servings per day, including dark green or yellow vegetables, citrus fruits or tomatoes. The methods by which vegetables are prepared are very important because when vegetables are overcooked most of the nutrients are lost. Cooked vegetables should be cooked quickly.

4. Four or more servings daily of breads and cereals. Enriched or whole-grain cereals have proved to be the best, not only for the bulk they add to the diet but also from the nutritional standpoint. White bread made from enriched flour has proved not as nutritionally acceptable as bread made from whole grains, such as pure whole wheat.

It is extremely important that nutritional requirements are met, both to keep the hard and soft tissues of the oral cavity healthy and for the general well-being of the individual patient.

8

Dental Disease

A healthy tooth is free from decay and has sound gums and supporting bone holding the tooth in place. What are the great enemies of healthy teeth? Until the age of twenty-five, decay is the most destructive dental process; after this age periodontal disease becomes the greater problem. In fact, more teeth are lost in adults because of periodontal disease than because of tooth decay.

Tooth decay is initiated by the action of bacteria on food left in the mouth by improper brushing and flossing techniques. As we must have food to survive, so must the bacteria that live in the mouth. In the twenty-four hours after we eat, we rid ourselves of the by-products from the food in our body. When bacteria are left in the mouth, the bacteria ingest the food there and give off a by-product called exudate.

The exudates given off by the bateria are acids that can start both the decay process and destructive periodontal disease. The bacteria can ingest some foods much more rapidly, such as simple carbohydrates (refined sugars, white flour, etc.). Thus, the decay and periodontal disease processes take place more rapidly. So, remember, bacteria are excreting acids in your mouth and in order to break this cycle of bacteria-food-acid formation, the teeth and mouth should be cleaned as soon as possible after the ingestion of food.

When the acids are formed, they attack the surface of the tooth enamel and then spread, attacking beneath the tooth surface. Usually, at this early stage the decay can be seen only by the dentist, with the aid of x-rays. When the decay has spread far enough, the enamel surface will collapse and you will be able to see the cavity. When a cavity can be seen by the naked eye, it has undermined the tooth surface with a good deal of decay and the underlying part of the tooth, called the dentin (which is much softer than the enamel), has been attacked. Once the dentin is attacked, and the decay continues to spread much more rapidly. At this point, the decay will not heal by itself but will need treatment by the dentist.

If not stopped by professional care, the decay can eventually reach the soft pulp tissue, which contains the nerves and blood vessels inside the tooth. An abscess may form. If this happens, not only can there be severe pain, but serious systemic problems can occur throughout the entire body because the infection has now been carried by the bloodstream and carried to other parts of the body. Endodontics would have to be performed or a tooth extracted at this point.

Not all people are vulnerable to decay and periodontal disease at the same rate. There is an unknown quantity called resistance that many individuals possess. It is the same characteristic that prevents some people from contracting tuberculosis and other diseases. There are individuals who have resistance to tooth decay and periodontal diseases, and the level of this resistance varies from one person to another; unfortunately the majority of people have none.

Without question, the major contributing factor to tooth decay and periodontal disease is *neglect*. In most instances, it cannot be blamed on heredity or water supply. Diet can have a significant effect, but the main contributing factor is neglect—not brushing and cleaning the teeth following the ingestion of any food. The accumulation of food debris, bacteria, and bacterial by-products is called plaque. Once plaque is allowed to remain for long periods of time it interacts again with bacteria and the environment of the oral cavity to form calcified deposits (calculus, or tartar).

VACCINE

Articles, in both the professional and lay press, have discussed a possible vaccine to prevent dental caries, or decay. Such vaccine for dental caries may be a fact in the future, but it is the belief of this author and many practitioners that, regardless of the vaccine, good oral hygiene on a daily basis by the patient will always be the most important factor in preventing dental caries, tooth decay, and periodontal disease.

One possible drawback to the development of a vaccine for caries is that individuals will become more relaxed in their hygiene and not brush their teeth, thinking that the vaccine will prevent decay. Consequently, the most prevalent oral disease in adults, periodontal disease, would probably become even more prominent. Periodontal disease, except in the cases of those few individuals who have rare systemic disease, exists in direct relation to the way patients care for their mouth by brushing and flossing conscientiously on a daily basis. Periodontal disease can only be prevented through a conscientious oral hygiene program performed by the patient each day.

PERIODONTAL DISEASE

Periodontal disease is not a disease that affects only old people. It can begin early in life, when the first tooth erupts from the gum, and can continue undetected for years. Almost half the people in the United States over fifty years old have lost teeth due to periodontal disease.

To maintain healthy teeth and gums, a daily program of oral hygiene *must* be followed. When your gums are healthy, they are firm, pink, and fit tightly against the teeth. Periodontal disease makes the gums appear red and swollen, and they bleed easily. Bad breath is another sign. The disease is caused by many kinds of bacteria and their interaction with foods; however, it is not contagious.

Bacteria of many different kinds are always present in the mouth. Most are harmless unless the mouth is not cared for properly. If these bacteria are left to grow undis-

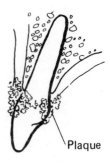
Plaque

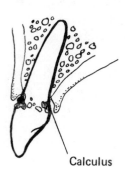
Calculus

turbed, they attach to the teeth and form communities, made up of millions of inhabitants. When the communities are formed at the edge of the gum, they produce pollutants that are absorbed by the gums, causing them to become red, swollen, and tender. When gums are healthy, the crevice, or ditch, around the teeth is shallow and does not contain many bacteria; however, if the space is deep, an accumulation can result, which can be a contributing factor to periodontal disease.

The bacteria not removed from the tooth surface continue to produce pollutants in the gums, leaving them soft and swollen, and this enlarges the space between the gums and teeth, leaving more space for the bacteria and making the teeth difficult to clean. The protective layer that normally covers the gum is destroyed, exposing the blood vessels. The gums bleed easily. The bacteria that cause this, once the disease reaches this stage, do not need the food we eat. They thrive on the nutrients and the tissue that fill and line the space. As long as the bacteria remain undisturbed, the disease continues to spread, often without discomfort, and can eventually attack and gradually destroy the bone that supports the teeth. This area gradually becomes larger, harboring more and more bacteria and pus. The larger the space becomes, the harder it is to clean; it is impossible to floss or brush these areas. At this point it becomes necessary to see a periodonist (gum specialist) for treatment.

If periodontal disease is not controlled, at some time in life all teeth may have to be removed because of the destructive process. A thorough examination by your dentist, plus periodontal probe and x-rays, is the best way to determine if you have periodontal disease. I have stated this previously in this book, but I shall emphasize it because of its importance: The dentist who does not use a periodontal probe, does not thoroughly examine your soft tissue, and does not discuss with you the problems of periodontal disease cannot correctly treat your mouth. He is like a man putting a new roof on a house while the foundation is collapsing.

Proper oral hygiene is important because the bacteria that attach to the teeth are soft and can be easily removed with floss and toothbrush on a daily basis, but if this accumulation is allowed to remain, it becomes hard and mineralized and has to be removed by the dentist or dental hygienist.

PERIODONTICS

Periodontics is the branch of dentistry that deals with the supporting structures of the teeth—the gums, the

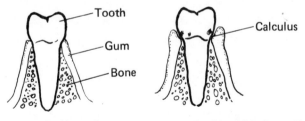

1. Normal   2. Gingivitis (gum disease)

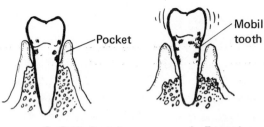

3. Periodontal disease   4. Excessive bone loss

bone, and surrounding tissues. Periodontics is one of the most important aspects of dentistry. As a house must have a good foundation to withstand the forces of time, so must the teeth have a good foundation to withstand the forces of mastication and to function in comfort and beauty for a lifetime.

There are several types of periodontal disease and extensive periodontal disorders that must be treated by a qualified periodontist. If your dentist tells you that you have a periodontal problem and need treatment and if the treatment seems to be complex, it might be advisable to seek the aid of a periodontist. For those who live in smaller communities, a periodontist is not always available, which means traveling to a larger city.

When periodontal disease is allowed to continue over a long period of time, the gum fibers connecting the gum to the teeth and the bone are eventually destroyed. The only way to correct this is with one of the many types of periodontal surgery.

Cost

Fees for periodontal treatment can range from $100 to $1,000, depending upon the type of treatment, the severity of the disease, and the method of treatment.

ENDODONTICS

Endodontics (root-canal therapy) was first recognized as a specialty in the mid-sixties. It has been used, however, to save teeth for over a hundred years. Many general practitioners are trained to perform most types of endodontics capably, but in multi-rooted teeth and difficult areas to treat, the patient should be referred to an endodontist.

Endodontics is usually necessary once the decay has found its way through the enamel and dentin to the pulp chamber. The bacteria invade this area and eventually destroy these tissues; the pulp chamber provides a ready haven for growth because it is dark, moist, and fertile. The bacteria colony grows, destroying the tissues in the pulp chamber. The bacteria, having no place else to go, find their way to the apex (root end) of the tooth where an abscess is formed by the body defenses in the bone. This created what is commonly known as an "abscess." The abscess is fed by the bacteria that are in the pulp chamber. Consequently, either the pulp chamber or the tooth must be removed. It is much wiser to save the tooth, if at all possible.

The pulp chamber is opened, cleaned out, and sterilized. It is then filled with an inert, sterile material, which

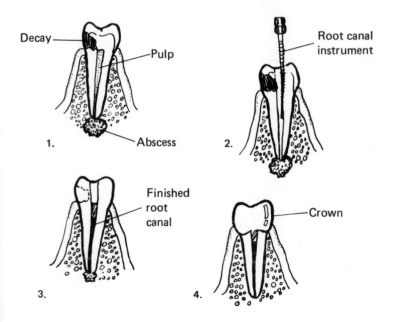

can be either gutta-percha, silver, or other material. A root canal can take from one to several appointments. It is one of the finest services that dentistry has to offer, because it allows teeth to be saved that would otherwise have to be extracted.

It is not true that once a tooth has had a root canal it will not decay. A tooth can also still develop periodontal disease. The only thing different about the tooth that has undergone endodontics is that it has no nerve impulse or blood vessel.

Although a tooth that has undergone a root canal is alive and well when supported by healthy periodontal tissue, it should usually have a crown because it will be more brittle.

Cost

- Single-rooted tooth $50 to $150
- Multi-rooted tooth $150 to $250
- Apicoectomy (removal of root end) $150 to $250

9

Children's Dentistry

Children's dentistry for many years has taken a back seat, not only in dentistry but also in some dental schools and in the view of some parents. Good dentistry should start with children at a young age.

Regrettably, many parents, even though they know their children have dental problems, neglect them. Many children would rather go to the dentist than suffer the discomfort of decayed and jagged teeth or unpleasant mouth odors. Their parents do not take them because they are suffering under the illusion "Why spend money when the children are going to lose these teeth?" Unfortunately, if they would only maintain their children's teeth and have them taken care of on a routine basis, it would in many instances save much dental pain for both the child and parent, and a great deal of expense later in life. Unfortunately, many dentist's share this belief and feel that not as much care is needed with primary as with permanent teeth.

A child's teeth should be cleaned and maintained just as if they were an adult's teeth because a child is going to have to keep these teeth from age three through twelve, *nine years of his life*. During this time, they enable the child to chew well, aiding in digestion, and they are important in the development of the jaw and face. The child should be taken to the dentist for the first time at approximately three years of age, when most children's deciduous teeth (baby teeth) have fully erupted into the arch.

Parents should be aware of sloppy work in children's dentistry. Whether it is a silver amalgam restoration, a stainless steel crown, a spacer, or a thumb-sucking appliance, regardless of what the dentist does for your child, it should be done with as much concern as if it were done for adult teeth.

SPACERS

One of the greatest dental crimes a parent can commit is to neglect replacing a deciduous (baby, or primary) tooth that has been lost or extracted. This replacement holds the space open where the tooth has been lost in the developing jaw so when it comes in it will have sufficient and proper room to erupt properly into the mouth.

When a baby tooth is lost and the space is not maintained the dynamic growth pattern of the jaw will cause the teeth to drift. This drifting of the teeth can cause a closing of the space, which will then prevent sufficient room for the adult tooth to erupt. This can cause serious problems that can only be corrected with orthodontics in years to come. It also causes the overlapping and crowding of teeth. Food becomes impacted, increasing the chances of

ERUPTION CYCLE

Deciduous Dentition

	Crown Completed		*Eruption*		*Root Completed*	
	Maxilla (Upper)	*Mandible (Lower)*	*Maxilla (Upper)*	*Mandible (Lower)*	*Maxilla (Upper)*	*Mandible (Lower)*
Central Incisors	1½ mo.	2½ mo.	9⅓ mo.	7½ mo.	1½ yr.	1½ yr.
Lateral Incisors	2½	3	11	13¼	2	1½
Cuspid	9	9	19½	19⅔	3¼	3¼
1st Molar	6	5½	15⅓	16	2½	2¼
2nd Molar	11	10	28	26½	3	3

Permanent Dentition

	Crown Completed		*Eruption*		*Root Completed*	
	Maxilla (Upper)	*Mandible (Lower)*	*Maxilla (Upper)*	*Mandible (Lower)*	*Maxilla (Upper)*	*Mandible (Lower)*
Central Incisors	4½ yr.	3½ yr.	7—7½ yr.	6—6½ yr.	10—11 yr.	8½—10 yr.
Lateral Incisors	5½	4—4½	8—8½	7¼—7¾	10—12	9½—10½
Cuspid	5½—6½	5½—6	11—12	9¾—10¼	12½—15	12—13½
1st Bicuspid	6½—7½	6½—7	10—11	10—10¾	12½—14½	12½—14
2nd Bicuspid	7—8½	7—8	10¾—11¼	10¾—11½	14—15½	14½—15
1st Molar	4—4½	3½—4	6—6⅓	6—6¼	9½—11½	10—11½
2nd Molar	7½—8	7—8	12¼—12¾	11¾—12	15—16½	15½—16½
3rd Molar	12—16	12—16	20½	20—20½	18—25	18—25

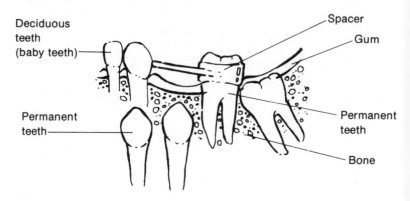

decay and periodontal disease. It may also cause gum problems that can be devastating later in life.

So the simple loss of a child's tooth should not be neglected.

Cost

Spacers can range from $45 to $90.

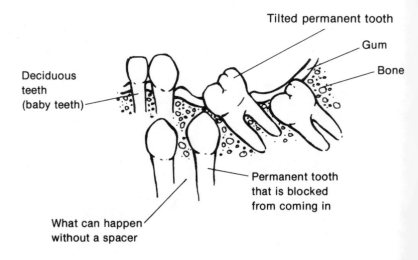

STAINLESS STEEL CROWNS

A child's tooth that is badly decayed and cannot be restored often must be crowned. It is foolish to crown this tooth by employing the conventional method used for crowning adult teeth. In most instances, precast stainless steel crowns are used. After the decay is cleaned out of the tooth and a sedative dressing placed in the tooth, the preformed stainless steel crown is cemented in place.

Cementing the crown helps protect the tooth from further decay and helps prevent the untimely loss of the tooth. The tooth will be exfoliated (come out of the mouth) at the proper time and be replaced by a permanent tooth.

Cost

A stainless steel crown is usually $25 to $50.

ANKYLOSIS

A high percentage of children do not lose their teeth at the proper time for reasons we do not know.

Some of these children experience what is called *anky-*

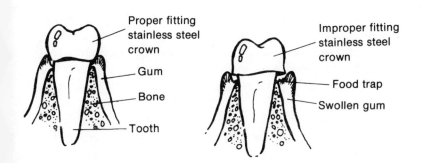

losis. The tooth becomes attached to the bone and is not lost in proper sequence. The teeth should then be extracted so that the proper eruption cycle can occur.

Ankylosis is not a common disorder, but it does occur often enough to be of concern.

INTERCEPTIVE ORTHODONTICS

Today there are many general dentists and pedodontists (children's dentists) who practice a type of dentistry called "interceptive orthodontics." This is when children are watched to determine whether their teeth are growing properly and following a normal eruption cycle. Certain procedures can be carried out by the dentist to intercept problems and correct them before more severe orthodontic problems manifest themselves. In many cases it is not possible to treat a case in this manner, and the child and the parents seek the counsel and guidance of a qualified orthodontist.

There are many things that a dentist can do today to prevent problems. He can aid the child in breaking harmful habits, such as tongue-thrusting (the pushing of the tongue against the front teeth) and thumb-sucking. The correction of these problems is one type of interceptive orthodontics.

Children's teeth should be checked for permanent teeth that never develop (congenital missing permanent teeth). When this occurs, and it is not uncommon, the parents should be aware of it as early as possible. In most instances, x-ray examinations can reveal this problem at an early age. Certain steps should be taken by the dentist to aid the child, if this happens.

If a child is unfortunate enough not to have a replacement tooth for a baby tooth, the baby tooth will often remain intact in the jaw until he is in his twenties or thirties. When it is eventually lost, it must be replaced by a bridge.

On occasion it may become necessary to reduce the crown of some of these baby teeth if they are to be maintained into adulthood. Some baby teeth are actually larger than the permanent teeth that replace them.

Cost

Interceptive orthodontic fees can range from $50 and up, depending upon the type of case.

FLUORIDATION

Fluoride has been proved effective against tooth decay when properly applied by either dentist or dental hygienist or when ingested orally in the water supply.

It has been known since the early thirties that fluoride can help reduce tooth decay. In a study on patients between thirteen and seventeen years of age, a single application of buffered stannous fluoride reduced caries 16 to 24 percent over a twelve-month period. When an 8 percent stannous fluoride solution was used on children and accompanied by good oral hygiene care, the results were even better. Studies done by the Dental Corps of the Canadian Air Force and United States Navy showed that stannous fluoride therapy was equally effective in adults and children.

Fluoride can be most effective against decay in children and adults, when properly used, in applications in the dental office, and in conjunction with the daily intake of fluoride in the water supply, and in dentifrices. Fluoride will make the teeth stronger and more resistant to tooth decay, but without proper oral-hygiene care on a day-today basis, it will not in itself prevent dental disease.It has also proved effective in certain types of tooth filling materials against the recurrence of decay.

Fluoride has been condemned because it is used in rat poison. This is true, but in rat poison it is used in large quantities. Chlorine is also used in certain rodent poisons, yet chlorine, in the proper amounts, has been used for hundreds of years in the purification of water supplies.

Fluoride in the water supply should be of number one concern to all individuals. Young children should have some sort of dietary fluoride, either in the water supply or added in vitamins. Of course, the dentist should be consulted, because if there is fluoride in the water it should not be more than one part per million. In those areas where there is stannuous fluoride in the water supply at percentages greater than this level, staining of the teeth can occur.

Cost

Fluoride treatment in a dental office ranges from $10 to $15.

10

Orthodontics

The orthodontist is thought of first as a dentist who straightens teeth; however, he also corrects bites and guides the proper development of facial bones. The psychological effects of going through life with crooked teeth can be devastating to a child as well as to an adult. What an orthodontist does for an individual is many times of greater psychological than physical benefit.

In years past, it was thought that orthodontics should not be attempted on children until they were twelve years old, or until after all the adult teeth were erupted. But, with the development of "interceptive orthodontics," that is, intercepting the problem before it really becomes serious, orthodontics is now started while the child is very young. Interceptive orthodontics can be properly practiced by the general dentist, or the pedodontist (children's dentist), or by the orthodontist himself.

There are several ways in which an orthodontist can treat maloccluded teeth: with fixed appliances (metal bands that are put around individual teeth and wired together) or with removable appliances. The latter can be quite successful when applied by a competent practitioner but it should be used only with minor tooth movement.

Have the orthodontist show you "before" and "after" models of previous cases he has treated, and have him give you a fixed fee for the treatment. Don't get in the trap of paying so much a month until the treatment is completed. I have known patients to go to an orthodontist for six or seven years. Other individuals with similar problems who have gone to an orthodontist with a fixed fee, have had the problem solved within two years. Be cautious. A special type of x-ray, called the cephalometric x-ray, which the orthodontist uses to determine the development of the head and face, must always be taken.

REMOVABLE ORTHODONTIC APPLIANCES

If the patient is interested only in having the front teeth look good, he might consider removable appliances. They are not suggested as a substitute for true orthodontics. In some instances where removable appliances are improperly used, periodontal damage can occur. This fact should be considered and discussed with a qualified orthodontist before treatment is undertaken.

Removable appliances come in many shapes, sizes, and designs. These appliances are used primarily to tilt and move teeth to give the patient a nice smile. They are referred to by some dentists as a "six-anterior appliance." That is, the six anterior (front) teeth that are normally seen when you smile and talk usually can be helped by using removable appliances.

Cost

The price for the removable orthodontic appliances can range from $65 to $225.

FULL ORTHODONTIC TREATMENT

It should be understood by the patient that in true orthodontics, which requires full banding, the orthodontist is attempting to do more than simply straighten the teeth or give the child a nice appearance. Here, not only the appearance of the patient, but also the growth and development of the face, and the establishment of a proper bite are taken into consideration. When the teeth come together properly the best periodontal condition possible can be maintained by the patient after treatment. The teeth can be kept clean, food will not impact between the teeth.

When straightening the teeth and correcting the bite are required for a patient, orthodontic bands should be the first consideration. The molar teeth, which have two, three, or more roots, usually require orthodontic bands in order to maintain the proper leverage and anchorage to move the teeth adequately without tilting them.

Cost

An average fee for most orthodontic treatments is from $1,000 to $2,000. Treatment can last from eighteen months to three years.

IMPROPER OCCLUSION

The word occlusion means coming together. When the teeth come together they are occluding. Malfunction of occlusion can result from   periodontal disease, which causes the shifting and drifting of teeth. When a person has extensive periodontal disease and surgery is performed to alleviate the problem, often times the bony support of the teeth is diminished. Because of this lessening of bony support, it becomes necessary to equilibrate (or adjust) the occlusion to take undue stress and strain off the individual teeth and supporting structures.

Improper occlusion can also be caused by attrition, which is the normal wearing away of teeth through years of normal use, or by congenital defects. If the latter is the case, treatment is best performed by an orthodontist.

There are several methods by which occlusal equilibration is performed. Generally it is accomplished by some method of marking the areas that are *not* coming together properly; then with the use of the high-speed "drill," portions of the teeth are ground away and reshaped in order that they will fit together better. Think of the occlusion as the cogs of a wheel coming together. If these cogs of the

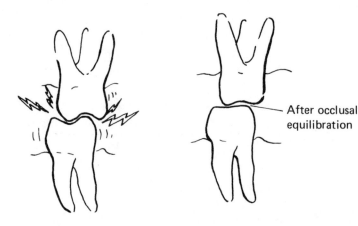

After occlusal
equilibration

Improper occlusion

wheel mesh properly, then the parts of the machine run properly. If they are out of alignment the machine will not run properly. The same thing is true with occlusal adjustment. In extensive cases, the patient is often referred to a periodontist to have the occlusal adjustment performed.

The treatment is also rendered in some instances to reduce temporomandibular joint pain. This is the joint where the lower jaw articulates with the skull. If teeth are out of alignment, it can cause pain in this joint, which is just below the ear. With proper occlusal equilibration, this can be corrected.

Cost

The cost of occlusal equilibration can range from $100 to $400.

NIGHT APPLIANCES

Night appliances are valuable for many patients. If the patient is aware of grinding the teeth (bruxism), a night appliance should be constructed.

Grinding the teeth can shake them and loosen them in their bony sockets. Continual shaking of a fence post will

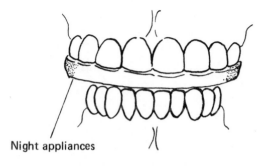

Night appliances

cause the ground to become loose, and the post can be removed from the soil. The same holds true for the supporting structures of the tooth that have become loosened.

Night appliances are easy to construct, and many adults, particularly in the middle years, require them. Patients usually adapt to night appliances quite readily. The appliance keeps the teeth from meshing together like cogs, thus preventing damage to the bony support of the teeth. When the lower jaw is moved, the teeth slide against the night appliance instead of grinding against the upper teeth.

Cost

The appliances range in cost from $80 to $150.

11

Restorative Dentistry

It is quite possible that the Etruscans introduced fixed dental bridge treatment to the Romans. Certain references to dental prosthesis for the restoration of mouths are found in the Roman Laws of the Twelve Tablets, which were written in 60-45 B.C. The first president of our country, George Washington, wore dentures. One set, we know, was made of wood. For centuries mankind has made an effort to develop a method of restoring missing teeth in order that individuals can function more comfortably. With the materials, experience, and equipment that are available today in dentistry, teeth can be restored and replaced, in most instances satisfactorily. But again, it is up to the dentist performing the procedures, and the patient in cooperation with the dentist, to realize the fulfillment of adequate dental care after the restoration of decayed and missing teeth.

SILVER AMALGAM ALLOY

Silver amalgam alloy is probably the most widely used and also the most abused of all dental restorative materials. In order for you to know you are receiving a satisfactory silver amalgam alloy, which is also called silver filling, amalgam filling, or alloy filling, the following should be noted:

1. After the tooth is prepared, the dentist should use a base in the bottom of the tooth that will act as an insulator.

2. The tooth should be thoroughly dried and kept dry, preferably by using a rubber dam (see below).

3. If it is a two-surface filling and a band has to be placed around the tooth, ask the dentist to let you see the post-operative x-ray so you can check to see that there is no overhang of the silver alloy, in other words that the alloy matches the proper contour of the tooth.

4. After the dentist has finished, you should note whether food gets in between the filling and the adjacent tooth. If this occurs, it has not been properly filled and the contact is open.

5. If the tooth feels high when you bite down, the filling must be adjusted before damage occurs to the tooth.

6. If the filling is rough, the dentist should polish the alloy in order to make the margins as smooth as possible, so they will not attract food debris and bacteria.

Silver amalgam alloy should not be called a permanent filling. There is nothing permanent in dentistry. The life of a silver filling is in direct proportion to how it is placed in the tooth and how the patient cares for his mouth on a daily basis. When there is adequate tooth structure left to hold the filling, the silver amalgam alloy may last many years. For a bucket to hold water, it must have all its sides. For a tooth to adequately hold a silver amalgam filling, it must have most of its sides left. A silver amalgam alloy does not have as much edge-strength (the capacity to resist fracture in thin sections) as other restorative materials.

A silver amalgam restoration should not be used for more than a three-surface filling, it should not be used because alloy breaks too easily. When too much tooth structure has been destroyed by decay, some sort of metal casting—an inlay, onlay, or crown restoration—should be used on the tooth.

Cost

The cost of a silver amalgam alloy can range from $10 to $30 per surface. Think of a tooth as a five-sided box, each side being a surface.

RUBBER DAM

The rubber dam is used by the dentist to isolate the tooth or teeth being treated and remove them as much as possible from the oral fluids of the mouth. The tooth should be kept as dry as possible. The rubber dam is nothing more than a piece of rubber with a hole punched in it. It is stretched until it will slip over the tooth. When the rubber is released, it forms a tight collar around the neck of the tooth and keeps the fluids of the mouth away. In most instances, it allows the dentist better access to the tooth. The rubber dam cannot be used in every procedure or in every instance of dental treatment, but when at all possible it should be used.

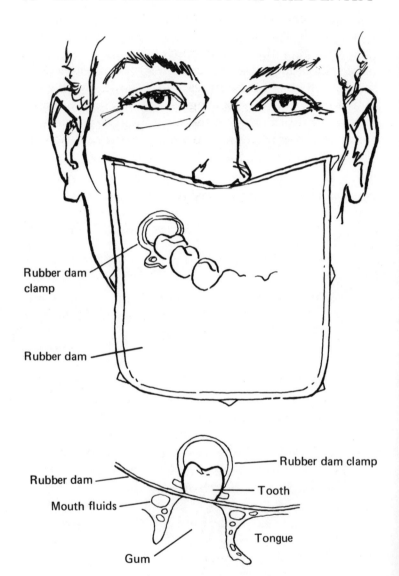

Rubber dam clamp

Rubber dam

Rubber dam clamp

Rubber dam

Tooth

Mouth fluids

Tongue

Gum

The rubber dam is used in almost all dental schools, but very few dentists use them once they are in practice, except for endodontics, for which it is imperative.

Use of a rubber dam is generally a sign of excellent dentistry and is one of the best ways to determine what kind of treatment you are receiving. If you go to a dentist and he uses a rubber dam for the majority of dental procedures, you may be fairly sure you are going to a meticulous, conscientious dentist.

SILVER AMALGAM ALLOY (WITH PINS)

Pins are much like the reinforcing steel that goes into concrete piers, bridges, or buildings. When a tooth is badly decayed and broken down, metal pins can be placed in the tooth. The pins are added support for the silver amalgam alloy.

Using pins with silver alloy can be an excellent method for restoring a tooth; however, there are several things to be cautious of. The tooth can become extremely sensitive because the pins are often placed adjacent to the pulp, which houses the nerve.

Pins, when properly used, can extend the life of a silver amalgam alloy and prevent the alloy from breaking. Many times a dentist will use pins and alloys to build up a tooth in order that there will be enough clinical crown

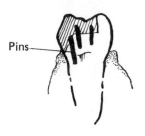

Pins

(that part of the crown visible in the oral cavity) left to place a gold crown casting over the tooth. Ask the dentist to let you see x-rays so you can see that the pins have not inadvertently been placed in the pulp chamber of the tooth.

Cost

The insertion of pins usually ranges from $15 to $40 plus the cost of the silver amalgam alloy.

COMPOSITE

Composite restoration material is a relatively new dental substance developed in the last decade. It has been useful in front teeth because it has the same natural color as a tooth. Although its primary use is in restoring cavities in the front teeth, it is also used for some back teeth. However, recent studies have shown that it should not be used in posterior (back) teeth that are used for chewing. Composites are also used in molar and bicuspid teeth on occasion, but they will not hold up there as long as other types of restorations.

If the dentist places the composite in the tooth with the use of a rubber dam, and all saliva is kept away from the tooth, you may feel secure that you are receiving better than average dental treatment. Composite restorations should be treated with an insulating base material to pre-

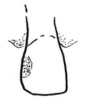
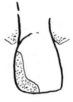
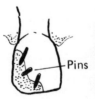

vent sensitivity to heat and cold and to prevent damage
the pulp of the tooth from the chemical change the composite undergoes as it hardens. No spaces should be left between the teeth to collect food debris after the tooth is restored and the filling should be polished so that there is no roughness to collect bacteria.

Composite restorations will stain in the mouths of heavy smokers, coffee drinkers, and tea drinkers.

Pins have been used in conjunction with composites in badly broken down anterior teeth, but the teeth will usually be weak, and the patient should be aware that they can break at any time. When this occurs, the teeth will have to be crowned.

Cost

Composite restorations can range from $15 to $25 a surface.

GOLD FOIL

Gold foil is a method of restoring a decayed area in a tooth with pure gold. The dentist manipulates gold foil in a well-prepared cavity, a small amount at a time, pressing it into place until the cavity is filled completely with gold. The filling is then shaped and polished.

Although gold foil is one of the oldest types of restoration in this day and age, with the modern material now available, it is seldom performed. The use of gold foil is difficult, slow, and expensive. If a dentist performs a gold foil procedure, he is usually a very excellent operator, but the patient must be prepared to pay.

Most people do not like gold foil because of its highly visible color and high cost.

Cost

A gold foil procedure can range from $50 to $100.

INLAYS/ONLAYS

Gold inlay or onlay is one of the better methods for restoring a tooth. Properly performed, an inlay replaces that portion of the tooth that has been destroyed by the ravages of decay, leaving the majority of the walls of the tooth still intact; the inlay fits in the tooth. An onlay is used when portions of the walls of the teeth are also destroyed. An onlay fits *on* the tooth, as the name implies, whereas the inlay fits *in* the tooth.

There are several methods used to construct the inlays/onlays, but usually the tooth is prepared, an impression is made, and from the impression, a die is made. The die is sent to a dental laboratory. The patient usually wears a temporary medicated filling until the restoration is ready to be placed in the tooth, at which time the temporary is removed, and the finished restoration is placed in or on the tooth.

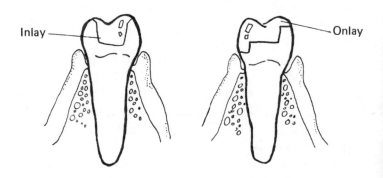

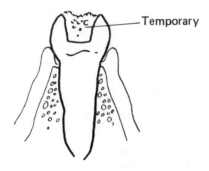

Temporary

Things to watch for:

1. Ask to see x-rays after the dentist has finished the treatment, to be assured that there are no overhanging margins.

2. The tooth should not be high when you close your teeth together. For example, you should not feel that you bite with this tooth first.

3. The contact should be tight, not allowing food debris to collect between the teeth, but you should still be able to pass dental floss between the teeth.

4. There should be no roughness to the touch of the finger or the tongue.

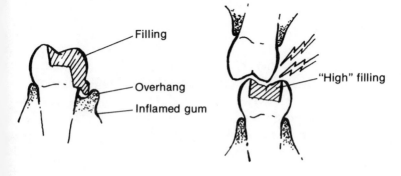

Filling

Overhang

Inflamed gum

"High" filling

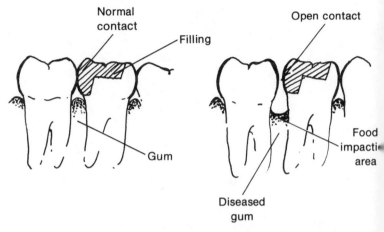

When your dentist takes an impression, make sure that it is not made with impression material that is mixed with water. There are some impression materials available that can be mixed with water that generally are not accurate enough to take a detailed final impression for gold work of any kind.

Cost

The average cost of an inlay, or onlay, is $160 to $250. This price may vary today because of the unstable price of gold.

CROWNS

Often, teeth that have been neglected for long periods of time cannot be restored using the conventional restorative materials such as silver amalgam alloy or composites. The tooth must then be crowned. The term crown refers to the fact that the crown completely covers the portion of the tooth above the gum. This process is sometimes called *capping*.

There are several types of crowns:

1. *The full crown* completely covers the tooth down to, and in many instances beneath, the edge of the gum line. Crowns can be made of gold alloy. They have been made of silver in the past. In some countries in Europe, they are made of cast stainless steel; crowns have been made of acrylic, but this should be used only for a provisional or temporary crown.

2. *The three-quarter crown* usually covers all of the tooth except for that portion seen when the patient is smiling or talking (the buccal, outside, portion of the tooth).

3. *The veneer crown* is a full crown with the visible part of the crown covered with a material that has the appearance and color of the tooth structure. One type

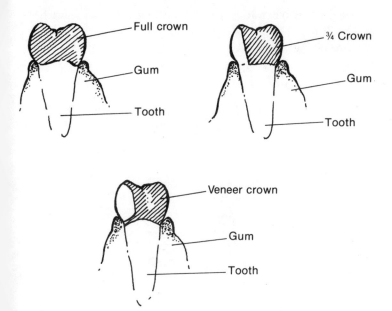

is the porcelain-on-gold crown. The porcelain is baked directly onto the gold. A special gold is used that can withstand the high heat required to bake the porcelain. This is one of the best types of restorations available, because the porcelain will not stain or become dark and unsightly under normal wear. Another type is the acrylic plastic veneer crown. This has a plastic on the visible portion of the gold crown. Unfortunately, plastic expands and contracts greatly, and absorbs the liquids in the mouth. Usually, in a matter of a few years this type of crown discolors and becomes unsightly. It will wear away under normal brushings, and chewing gum sticks to it.

The process involved in making a crown is as follows:

1. The decay is removed from the tooth.

2. If the tooth is badly decayed, the tooth may have to be built up. This building-up can be done with alloys or a combination of alloy pins, or with a post that is cast. It gives more surface area to the tooth, so the final crown can be seated.

3. Once the tooth is prepared, the gum tissue is treated so that a good, accurate impression can be made around

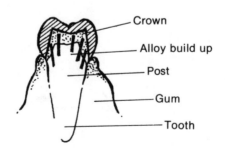

the tooth. The impression is sent to the laboratory, where the crown is constructed.

4. The dentist then makes a temporary crown.

The patient should exhibit a great deal of concern over the temporary crown. It should not be a shell crown. Shell crowns are bought from dental supply houses and only come in a number of commercial sizes. They cannot be formed to fit the tooth accurately, and as a result gingival, or gum, irritation occurs. If a shell crown is left on the tooth for a long period of time, irreversible damage can be done to the gum tissue.

Such damage can also result from a crown cast and made by a dental laboratory, if it is not properly contoured. The contact should fit snugly against the adjacent tooth in order to prevent food impaction between the teeth. The temporary crown is usually seated with some sort of medicated cement to help prevent the tooth from being sensitive while the patient is waiting to receive the final crown.

Regardless of the type of crown that is inserted, there are several things the patient should be aware of: (1) If the crown seems high when biting (the patient is aware of hit-

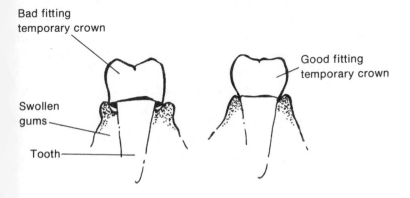

ting the crowned tooth first), then the patient should tell the dentist, and the tooth should be placed in proper occlusion. This condition, known as "prematurity," if allowed to remain, not only can be uncomfortable but can cause permanent tooth damage and damage to the supporting structures. (2) The contacts of the tooth should be firm and fitted tightly to the adjacent teeth so that food does not impact between the teeth during eating. The fit should not be so snug that dental floss cannot pass through readily. (3) The crown should be highly polished so that rough surfaces will not aid in the accumulation of plaque and bacteria. (4) The contour of the tooth should be such that as the patient chews, food does not in time do irreversible damage to the gum tissue. (5) The patient should ask to see an x-ray of the crown following insertion to make sure there are no overhanging margins to trap food and possibly cause further decay.

It is not unusual procedure on a badly broken-down tooth for a dentist to do a minimum amount of preparation on the tooth and cover the tooth with a provisional or temporary stainless steel crown. This crown is seated with a sedative cement to try to keep the tooth from being sensitive and suffering possibly permanent pulp damage.

If a tooth is extremely sensitive to hot and cold following insertion of the temporary crown, and if this sensitivity lasts more than a week or ten days, the patient should inform the dentist. There are several dental chemicals and medications available to the dentist that he can use on the prepared tooth to reduce the sensitivity. Often, however, it is necessary to remove the crown and coat it with a calcium hydroxide base or a zinc oxide eugenal preparation. Most teeth that are well-prepared and have a crown placed on them are sensitive for a day or so afterwards, but generally this condition goes away.

Cost

- A full-cast gold crown approx. $150
- A full-cast plastic veneer crown approx. $170
- A porcelain-on-gold crown approx. $200 to $300
- A three-quarter crown approx. $150

POSTS

To restore a tooth that has been badly neglected or accidentally injured, it is often necessary to use a post. The tooth must first have a root canal (endodontic procedure) in order to save the tooth. After the root canal is completed, the post is inserted deep into the pulp chamber of the tooth to anchor it and form a proper seat for the crown.

Decisions about what type of post is required are generally made by the dentist. There are several things about a post that the patient should determine when he sees the postoperative x-rays. The post should go deep into the root of the tooth. It should not extend out the side of the

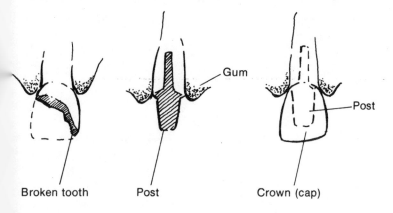

Broken tooth   Post   Gum   Post   Crown (cap)

tooth. And the tooth should not be sensitive after the post is placed in it.

Generally they are cast out of some kind of noncorrosive metal and cemented in place. Silver alloys with pins are occasionally used instead of posts; however, they are usually not as substantial as the posts. The type of post used is generally determined by which tooth requires it. For a single-rooted tooth, a post can often be constructed with pins, alloys, or composite restoration material. With posterior teeth it is often times necessary to cast a post, since they are multi-rooted.

Cost

Posts generally cost from $80 to $120, depending on the type used and the conditon of the tooth.

IMPLANTS

Many individuals, particularly those who suffer the discomfort of lower dentures, have hoped that implants would enable them to have comfort once again. Implants, however, should be considered as still experimental. They have been successful in a limited number of cases in which they are used in conjunction with remaining natural teeth. An extremely poor success record has been demonstrated for implants when there are no natural teeth remaining in the dental arch.

Implants generally fall into three categories:

Category 1: This is called the osteos implant. The tissue is opened up, the bone is exposed, and an impression is made of the bone. Then an implant is made that fits over the bone and is secured to it. The tissue is placed back over the implant. A male post is left extending

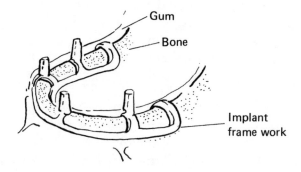

Gum

Bone

Implant frame work

through the tissue, then a female attachment is secured to the appliance for stabilization.

Category 2: The most popular type of implant is the *blade implant* in which an incision is made through the tissue into the bone. A groove is cut into the bone and the implant inserted. This fixed type of implant has had little success even when properly inserted and used in conjunction with natural teeth and has fallen into disre-

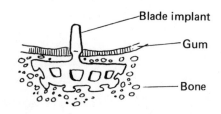

Blade implant

Gum

Bone

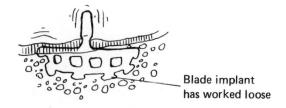

Blade implant has worked loose

pute. The body of the implant must be inserted completely beneath the bone. If it begins to become loose at all, it must be removed, because *this can be highly destructive to the bone.*

Category 3:   This fixed type of implant, called a *"carbon implant,"* is performed by placing a vitreous carbon implant in the bone and then screwing a post into the carbon implant. Even though this has proven to be the most successful type of implant, it has not been completely reliable.

Implants are not 100 percent successful, and many factors should be considered before implants are inserted. The general condition and health of the individual, the density and amount of bone present, the location of the implant (it is usually more successful in the lower jaw because of the density of the mandibular bone), the type of dental appliance to be constructed over the implant, the care that the individual gives his mouth as far as oral hygiene is concerned, and the way the implant is inserted—all affect the success of this procedure. Despite experimental work on both types of implants, neither can yet be recommended as 100 percent effective.

The patient should be aware of the failure rate of implants. There is always a possibility an implant will have to be removed sometime in the following years. Most dental researchers feel that nothing should be promised to the patient about the longevity of implants.

Cost

- Osteo implant   up to $1,500
- Blade implant $100/$200 up to $900
- Carbon implant   approx. $300

12

Prosthesis

Prosthetics is the dental specialty concerned with the artificial replacement of missing teeth. It is hoped that after reading this book, no one will have to suffer the pain, the discomfort, the odors, the sores, and the embarrassment of wearing full dentures. A great deal of care should always be given to the natural dentition in order to prevent the loss of any teeth. If your dentist is not primarily concerned with saving natural teeth, find another dentist. Unfortunately, teeth are lost either through neglect or accident. If this happens it is important to replace the missing teeth as soon as possible. The ways they can be replaced are numerous.

FULL DENTURES

The entire complement of teeth is replaced with denture plates. Denture teeth can be made of either plastic or porcelain. The base, which is the gum-colored material that supports the teeth and rests on the patient's natural gum tissue, is usually plastic, though it can be cast out of precious metal, such as gold. When dentures are being constructed, more than one impression should be made. Custom impression trays should be made of the patient's mouth. A "snap" impression should never be used as the final one. Dentures are difficult enough in themselves to wear, and with just one impression, the probability of a proper fit is very poor.

The use of a face bow should also help to ensure a better fit.It helps the laboratory to duplicate the bite more accurately, by measuring the relative position of the jaws. Its use by a dentist is a sign that you are getting quality dentistry.

Cost

• Full dentures   Lower—$185 to $300
                                     Upper—$185 to $300

IMMEDIATE DENTURES

If a person must have dentures, the most acceptable way to construct them is to take the impression before all the teeth are removed, then place the dentures in the mouth immediately following the removal of the last tooth. In most instances, people who have immediate dentures adapt to them more easily than if they have all their teeth extracted and dentures constructed sometime later.

Cost

• Immediate dentures   Lower—$250 to $350
                                     Upper—$250 to $350

REMOVABLE PARTIAL DENTURES

When some of the teeth are missing, they can be replaced with a removable partial denture. This type of appliance can be removed by the patient, cleaned, and replaced in the mouth. The removable partial denture can be made in many ways, but several factors should be understood about this appliance. The denture should be removed several times a day and cleaned thoroughly. Bacteria, food debris, and fungus accumulate underneath it, which can be very destructive to the soft tissues of the mouth and to the teeth that support the partial.

The teeth around which any clasp or removable denture rests, should be brushed more often than normal, because bacteria and food debris can also accumulate underneath the clasp. If not cleaned thoroughly, this is an excellent area for the incubation of bacteria and the formation of the destructive acids that cause tooth decay. It is not uncommon to find a ring of decay underneath the clasp of the tooth, and many dentists will recommend that crowns be placed on these abutment teeth to prevent this.

Another problem is a condition called *slow forceps*. This refers to the fact that the clasps that fit around the teeth, through years of wear and friction on the teeth and the torque that is applied to the teeth, can eventually cause these teeth to be lost.

Despite the problems, partials are generally more satisfactory than full dentures.

Cost

• Partial dentures   Upper—$225 to $350
                                         Lower—$225 to $350

OVERDENTURES

An overdenture is usually constructed for the lower jaw, but in some instances it is made for the upper jaw. Dentists have known since they first began to make artificial teeth for individuals that generally the upper denture will be quite successful, because in most people, with the greater surface area available, there is more suction. The lower denture is more often than not unsuccessful because of the attachment of the tongue and muscles and the narrow ridge.

To make the overdenture, two or more lower teeth are saved to attach the denture to and thus maintain some type of stability. In the past, when the teeth were so badly broken down this was impossible. In recent years, however, a method has been utilized for making overdentures when the two or more remaining teeth are not sound. If there is periodontal involvement, it is treated first, then root canals are performed on the teeth, and posts are placed in them. These posts protrude above the gum and fit into female attachments in the underside of the denture, making it much more stable.

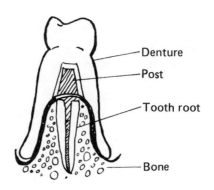

Cost

For each tooth that is used under the overdenture, the cost of the denture increases approximately $200 to $300. The comfort and function of the overdenture, as compared to ordinary dentures, is well worth the extra expense.

UNILATERAL, OR SPIDER, PARTIALS

The unilateral partial, which is referred to by dentists as the spider partial, is probably the most dangerous of all dental appliances. It is small and can be swallowed. If the teeth can accommodate a spider partial, they usually can accommodate a fixed bridge, which is a much better dental appliance.

Cost

The spider partial will vary in cost according to the number of teeth replaced. The average cost is $65 to $200. This is one type of dental treatment *that should never be considered.*

FLAPJACK PARTIALS

The flapjack partial is usually all acrylic (plastic). It is used often as a temporary partial following the extraction of teeth to hold the space until the healing process has

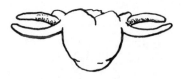

"Spider" partial

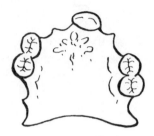

Flapjack partial

been completed. It is also used in children and adolescents as a provisional appliance to replace missing teeth until the mouth is more fully developed. Later, a more conventional type of dental appliance can be constructed.

The all-acrylic appliance should never be used as a final appliance. Unfortunately, many people are sold flapjack partials without being told they are considered a temporary restoration.

Cost

The cost should not exceed approximately $85 to $150.

CLASPS

A clasp is a metal attachment that holds a partial in place.

They can be made in two ways. Half-clasps are nothing more than bent, stainless steel wires, which are bonded into the body of the plastic partial. This gives little or no support to the partial but simply helps make the partial more stable in the mouth.

Cast clasps, which fit the teeth much more precisely, and also have a rest that helps prevent the partial from pressing against the gum tissue, are much more accepta-

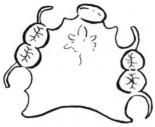

Flapjack partial
with half clasp

ble. Partials with half-clasps *should only be considered temporary partials.*

Cost

The cost of a flapjack partial with half-clasps is approximately $150.

CAST PARTIAL

The best removable partial denture, if you have to have a partial, is the cast partial. The entire partial is cast from either gold or one of the chromelike metals. The partial can be entirely metal, or the clasp and the body of the partial can be metal and the areas that are to hold the artificial teeth (saddle areas) can be made of plastic to give a more natural appearance when you are smiling and talking.

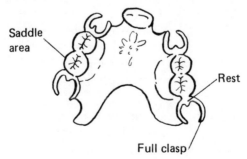

Saddle area

Rest

Full clasp

This type of partial, when properly constructed, can be of great service. The partial must be kept immaculately clean at all times to prevent decay of natural teeth and the development of periodontal disease.

Cost

This type of partial is usually in the price range of $200 to $300.

SWING LOCK PARTIALS

The swing lock, or stabilization, partial is used in a mouth that has had an excessive amount of bone loss around the teeth, causing the teeth to become mobile. The swing lock is hinged like a gate. When the partial is placed in the mouth, it is locked in position in order to support the remaining teeth firmly and keep them from undergoing extreme stress during the chewing of food.

Swing lock partials are used in some instances in periodontal therapy when teeth are loose. The locking arm of the partial acts as a splint to make the teeth more stable. Sometimes no artificial teeth are used in conjunction with this type of appliance.

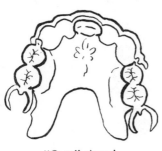

"Gate" closed

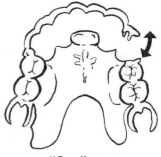

"Gate" open

Cost

The fee for this type of partial should be $300 to $400.

PRECISION PARTIALS

Precision partials are used in conjunction with cast crowns. This is accomplished by crowning the abutment teeth and constructing female attachments in the crown to hold the partial.

The partial is constructed with high precision male attachments that fit into these female attachments, holding the partial in place. The partial is made in conjunction

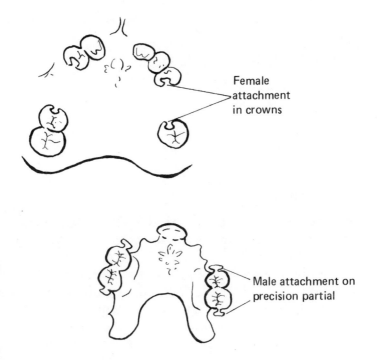

Female attachment in crowns

Male attachment on precision partial

with crowns and fixed bridges. It is considered the "Cadillac" of removable partial dentures.

Cost

It is difficult to give an average fee for such a partial. There are so many variables, such as the number of teeth replaced and the number of attachments. But, precision partials could cost as much as $1,000, not counting the crown that the partial attaches to.

Five Things To Look For To Determine If A Partial Fits Properly

1. It should not cause the teeth to which it is attached to be sore.

2. The partial should not cut into the tissue or cause sore spots.

3. There should be no rough edges.

4. The partial should be constructed in such a way that it does not trap food.

5. It should not press against the tissue in such a way that is causes redness or irritation.

FIXED PARTIALS

A fixed partial is more acceptable than a removable partial denture. It involves the replacement of teeth in such a manner that they are fixed in place and cannot be removed by the patient. The abutment teeth (the teeth that support and hold this bridge in the mouth) are generally covered with a full crown or three-quarter crown. The missing teeth are replaced with artificial teeth (pontics). These are soldered (welded) together to the crowns of the abutment teeth to form the bridge of the fixed prosthesis.

Several factors should be understood by the patient before he undertakes to subject himself to a fixed prosthesis:

1. The supporting structure of the remaining teeth must be extremely healthy. There should be adequate bone to support the roots. The roots should be situated deep within the bone in order to give the best support possible for the bridge.

2. If the bone is weak or the roots of the teeth are short and rounded, unwonted pressure can be applied to these teeth and cause further damage and their eventual loss.

3. If a three-unit bridge (one that has an abutment tooth on either side of the artificial tooth)is placed in the mouth, then two teeth are now supporting and working for three teeth.

4. The artificial teeth should always be narrow in order to reduce their chewing surface and reduce the stress on the abutment teeth.

5. The artificial teeth should be adapted so that the area where they rest against the gum tissue can be easily cleaned and maintained by the patient.

6. The fixed bridge should not have prematurities (irregular surfaces) and should not feel high when the patient bites and chews.

7. The contact between the abutment and the adjacent tooth must be tight.

8. There should be no overhang on the crowns that cover the abutment teeth.

9. There should be no roughness. The bridge should be smooth and clean.

Special instructions should always be given to the patient by the dentist or his assistants. These bridges must be taken care of much more vigorously than natural teeth. They should be brushed and cleaned with a dental floss around the bridge. Special threaders should be given to the patient by the dentist or his assistants so that the floss can be used underneath the artificial teeth.

TYPES OF FIXED BRIDGES

Fixed bridges—excellent appliances for replacing missing teeth—can be constructed in many ways. They can be fully cast metal or acrylic. Either the outside portion of the teeth that will be apparent or the whole bridge can be covered with porcelain or plastic. (Porcelain will usually last longer than plastic.)

When the whole bridge is cast of metal and completely covered with porcelain, this is called a full coverage, or porcelain-on-gold, bridge. Where only the visible surface is covered, it is called a veneer bridge. These covered bridges are usually the most aesthetically pleasing and are also usually the most expensive type of restorations.

An acrylic bridge should be used only as a temporary to be worn while the permanent bridge is being constructed. I have seen many patients who were told that they were permanent-type bridges. There is really nothing permanent in dentistry and certainly not in acrylic.

Your dentist should discuss with you the various types of bridges and facings. He should tell you what he recom-

Full gold
bridge
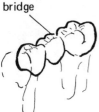

Veneer
bridge
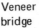
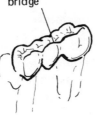

Full coverage
bridge
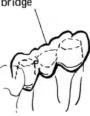

mends as the best choice of treatment in your particular case.

Do not, under any circumstances, ever tolerate:

1. A rough bridge

2. An unsightly bridge

3. A mismatched color bridge

4. A bridge that feels high

5. A bridge that traps food particles

6. A bridge that constantly has an odor or bad taste

7. A bridge that feels loose

Cost

Fixed bridges are usually priced by the *unit*. A unit represents one tooth; a three-unit bridge consists of the two abutment teeth and the tooth that is being replaced.

1. A fully cast bridge will be approximately $150 per unit.

2. A porcelain veneer bridge costs approximately $250 to $300 per unit.

3. A full coverage porcelain-on-gold bridge is $300 per unit.

4. An acrylic veneer bridge is approximately $200 per unit.

THE THIMBLE, OR TELESCOPIC, BRIDGE

The abutment teeth that are going to support the bridge are first prepared and then covered with a thin casting of gold. This covering, called a thimble, or telescope, is itself prepared and the bridge installed on top of it. This is an excellent type of restoration, but it must be understood that the thimbles will increase the cost of the bridge as much as $60 to $150 each.

Fixed bridges by nature undergo a certain amount of torque (turning or twisting). When a thimble is used with a fixed bridge, torque is less of a problem. If the bridge does work loose from the abutment, there will usually be no decay underneath the abutment crown to the soft underlying dentin, because it is covered by the thin layer of gold. The thimble cannot be used on all teeth because

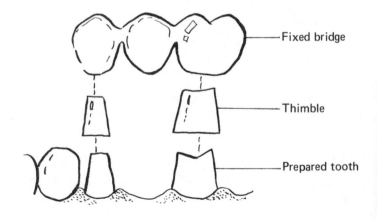

of the general anatomy of the tooth crown. With short, flat-crowned teeth, there is not enough room to install the thimble and bridge.

PRECISION BRIDGE

The precision fixed bridge is similar to the precision partial denture. The teeth are prepared and crowns are placed over them. Precision female attachments are made in these crowns. The male attachments are cast into the bridge. These can be used only when the patient fully understands that the abutment teeth must be given proper care. The gum tissue and bone around the tooth must be kept in excellent condition.

Cost

The attachments usually increase the price of the bridge approximately $100 to $200.

SPLINTS

The term *splint* refers to restoring the entire dental arch of the mouth. It is a bridge that generally takes in a

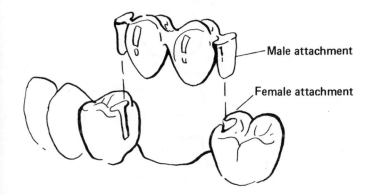

Male attachment

Female attachment

number of teeth. In many instances it does not replace missing teeth but simply ties loose teeth together to prevent them from being further loosened by normal mastication or grinding of the teeth. Teeth are splinted for the same reason that a broken arm is—so that it cannot be moved.

Generally, splints are performed on teeth that have extensive periodontal destruction (pyorrhea). The bone has become diseased and weakened around the teeth allowing them to become mobile. They must be tied together in order to prevent further destruction of bone around the teeth in the normal biting and chewing process.

Cost

The cost of splints can range from $200 a unit to $300 a unit (each tooth or tooth replacement represents a unit).

13

Things You Can Do to Receive Better Dentistry

The dentist-patient relationship is a very close relationship. Those individuals who have proper attitudes about dentistry usually receive better dental care. A patient who is unruly, aggressive, and demanding is going to be one that the dentist wants to get rid of and get out of the dental chair as quickly as possible. The treatment will be done as quickly as possible and because of this the patient may not receive as good dental treatment and care as he would have with a better attitude. Never say to the dentist, because dentists get tired of hearing it, "How much I hate coming to the dentist." Try telling the dentist how grateful you are that there is someone like him available to take care of your dental needs and make you comfortable. Everyone likes to be praised.

Don't be afraid to ask the dentist any question about the procedures he is performing. If there is any pain or discomfort be sure and tell him about it; don't try to be a martyr. Those individuals who prefer to have their dental treatment performed without dental anesthesia place a great psychological strain on the dentist since he is aware that he is hurting them.

1. Be on time for your appointment

2. Don't cancel. If you have to cancel, give two or three days notice, if possible—give your dentist an opportunity to fill up his valuable time. When you have a dental appointment and have to wait more than ten minutes, raise hell with the dentist. Your time is valuable, too. You should not have to wait.

3. Don't put an aspirin on an aching tooth.

4. If you have a medical or physical problem, be sure to inform your dentist.

5. Don't squirm in the chair.

6. Don't constantly pull your head aside.

7. Sit with your arms folded in your lap or on the armrests of the chair, not across your chest and not behind your head.

8. A woman should not wear a fancy hairdo; it makes it impossible for the patient to be comfortable in the dentist chair and difficult for the dentist to properly treat her.

9. Don't smoke in the dental treatment room. They are usually small rooms, and the air can become offensive to the dentist, the dental assistant, and other patients.

The presence of oxygen units in dental offices also makes smoking dangerous.

10. Don't rush the dentist. Don't ask him to hurry, you are the one who will suffer in the long run with sloppy dentistry. If the treatment the dentist is performing for you requires that something go to the dental laboratory, don't make a request that it be back early. This can only end in shoddy dentistry. Give your dentist plenty of time to do the dental treatment.

11. Accept appointments when it is convenient for the dentist to see you, because generally you will be scheduled when there are fewer patients and he has more time to treat you. If you insist on seeing him at the same time everybody else wants appointments, which is usually late in the afternoon, you may wind up getting the quick treatment.

12. Always demand that your dentist tell you how much the treatment is going to cost, but don't try to get your dentist to begin compromising on fees, because then he will be forced to begin *compromising on treatment*.

13. Don't ask the dentist to perform the most inexpensive form of treatment; generally this is the most costly in the long run. For instance, if a tooth is badly decayed and broken down, the dentist may suggest an inlay or a crown. If you insist that he try to fill it with a silver amalgam alloy, the silver alloy cannot withstand the force of biting and chewing. If it breaks you will have to have a root canal and a crown to save the tooth.

14. If after you go to your dentist and he tells you what you need you are still unsure, don't hesitate to ask him to send your records to someone else and get another

opinion, not just from a standpoint of trying to get the same treatment at a lower fee, but to see if the treatment that he recommends is basically sound. However, don't expect when you go to the second dentist that the treatment will be exactly the same. The education, the age of the dentist at the time he was educated, postgraduate training—all cause some variation. No two dentists are alike and no two dentists review most cases alike.

15. Pay for your dentistry promptly. What kind of treatment do you think you will receive if you owe a bill of many months' standing? Though we like to tell ourselves that this should not affect the dentist's attitude, remember a dentist is only human.

16. The dentist is not only available to serve mankind, he is also a businessman. If you have a complaint about the dentistry you receive, don't complain to other people. Go back to your dentist first. Give him an opportunity to either explain the situation or to straighten out the problem. If you get no satisfaction from him, then your first choice should be to write to the dental society to which he belongs—whether is it local, state, or national. If this is of no satisfaction, then there are always legal means. However, nearly all misunderstandings can be avoided by simply discussing the problem with your dentist. Most dentists are perfectly willing to work out all difficulties.

17. Go for your routine dental appointments every six months, or when the dentist advises. Have your teeth scaled and cleaned. You will find that this reduces your dental expenses in the long run. It makes the dentist aware that you are interested in your oral

health, and he becomes more interested in helping you. People who are very neglectful of their mouths and show little or no interest in taking care of them, sometimes get disinterested treatment. Why should the dentist break his back trying to give you the best treatment possible when you will not make the effort to take care of your own teeth. The dentist alone cannot maintain your dental health—he must have your cooperation.

Following these rules will not only provide better dentistry, but your dentist will be more inclined to be of help when an emergency arises. A dentist hates to hear a patient call, wanting to be seen immediately for a toothache he has had for two or three weeks. When you do have an urgent problem, make sure it is an emergency and not something that you finally decided is an emergency after weeks of discomfort.

HABITS THAT HARM

Finally, there are a few habits which which send many people to the dentist. If you can avoid them it will help to cut down on the dentistry you need.

1. The gnashing or clenching of teeth, called bruxism, is harmful. An effort should be made to find the stress and tension that create this problem. In the meantime, a bruxing appliance (night appliance) should be worn.

2. Chewing on pencils exerts unnatural force on teeth and can cause them to become loose. Biting or chewing a pipe can cause the same problem.

3. Tongue-thrusting in children (pushing the tongue forward when the child swallows) applies pressure on

the back of the front teeth, which can cause them to protrude.

4. Thumb-sucking puts abnormal pressure on teeth that can cause the upper teeth to protrude and the lower teeth to incline inward.

5. Sucking or biting the cheek can cause malocclusion problems.

6. Opening bobby pins with the teeth can cause breaking away of the edge of the teeth and unsightly notches.

7. Sucking on lemons or any fruit that is heavy in citric acid has an abrasive effect and can cause deterioration of the enamel.

8. Smoking is an unnatural habit. It is bad for the general body, for the teeth, and the gums. It stains the teeth, making them unsightly. It coats gums and teeth, forming a rough surface on the teeth that makes it easier for the bacteria to attach themselves.

9. Breathing through the mouth has a drying effect on the teeth and prevents the teeth from being bathed in the neutralizing saliva, causing high instances of decay.

10. Chewing ice can cause breaking of the teeth, chipping of the enamel, and in some instances, the splitting of teeth.

11. Carrying nails and tacks in the mouth not only raises the risk of swallowing them, but, like bobby pins, they can crack teeth and injure gums.

Index

Page numbers in *italics* indicate illustrations.

111